Table of Contents

Practice Test #1 ....
    Practice Questions 4
    Answers and Explanations 33
Practice Test #2 61
    Practice Questions 61
    Answers and Explanations 91

Practice Test #1

Practice Questions

Section Description: Eggers Case Questions (Questions 1-11)

Samantha Eggers is an 18-year-old patient with end-stage kidney disease. She has begun automated peritoneal dialysis (APD) (also called continuous cycling peritoneal dialysis [CCPD]).

1. Ms. Eggers has become increasingly withdrawn, answering in monosyllables and exhibiting a flat affect. The patient may benefit most from
    a. change to hemodialysis.
    b. psychological counseling.
    c. social worker.
    d. spiritual support.

2. If Ms. Eggers is using APD with a long day dwell, icodextrin could be used
    a. as the "last bag option."
    b. for the first nighttime cycle.
    c. for all the nighttime cycles.
    d. for no cycles because it is not appropriate for CCPD.

3. Because Ms. Eggers has not been adhering to a healthy diet, the physician orders amino acid–based dialysate solution for nutritional supplementation. This solution should be used for
    a. all dwells.
    b. all nighttime dwells.
    c. one 4- to 6-hour dwell daily.
    d. one time only.

4. Which of the following is a water-soluble vitamin that should be supplemented for Ms. Eggers?
    a. Vitamin D.
    b. Vitamin A.
    c. Vitamin K.
    d. Vitamin B9.

5. If Ms. Eggers receives calcium carbonate as a phosphate binder, how much calcium is usually contained in the PD solution used for dialysis?
    a. 2 to 2.5 mEq/L.
    b. 3 mEq/L.
    c. 3.5 mEq/L.
    d. 4 mEq/L.

6. When teaching Ms. Eggers about peritoneal transport and absorption of fluid per the lymphatics, the patient should understand that peritoneal fluid is usually absorbed at the rate of
   a. 1 to 2 mL/min.
   b. 2 to 3 mL/min.
   c. 3 to 4 mL/min.
   d. 4 to 5 mL/min.

7. If Ms. Eggers reports a break in sterile technique that may have resulted in contamination of the peritoneal cavity, the nurse expects that the immediate response will be to
   a. institute preventive antimicrobial treatment.
   b. wait and watch for up to 12 hours.
   c. obtain a specimen of peritoneal fluid for culture.
   d. wait and watch for up to 48 hours.

8. If Ms. Eggers tests positive for peritonitis, which method of administration of antibiotics is generally recommended?
   a. Oral.
   b. Intravenous.
   c. Intraperitoneal.
   d. IM/Subcutaneous.

9. Because of changes in permeability of the peritoneum resulting from peritonitis, Ms. Eggers should be carefully monitored for
   a. hyperglycemia.
   b. hypoglycemia
   c. hypocalcemia.
   d. hypercalcemia.

10. Nystatin is recommended along with antibiotics during treatment for bacterial peritonitis in which patients undergoing peritoneal dialysis?
    a. All patients.
    b. Patients with symptoms of fungal infection.
    c. Patients in centers with high baseline rates of fungal infections.
    d. No patients, as nystatin is contraindicated in dialysis patients.

11. As Ms. Eggers is being treated for peritonitis, fibrinous clots develop in the peritoneal fluid. Which of the following treatments does the nurse expect?
    a. Addition of heparin to the dialysis solution.
    b. Irrigation of the catheter between dwells.
    c. More frequent exchanges.
    d. Temporary hemodialysis.

Section Description: Brock Case Questions (Questions 12 -20)

> *James Brock is a 46-year-old man with acute kidney injury following an automobile accident that resulted in blood loss, abdominal injuries, and a fractured pelvis. Because his kidneys are not functioning adequately, the patient requires temporary hemodialysis.*

12. Mr. Brock has a non-tunneled temporary hemodialysis catheter (NTHC) inserted into the femoral vein. Which of the following is a serious complication of femoral catheterization?
    a. Central venous stasis.
    b. Pneumothorax.
    c. Arrhythmia.
    d. Retroperitoneal hemorrhage.

13. In order to reduce the risk of complications, when an NTHC is inserted into the femoral vein, the practitioner should utilize
    a. anatomic landmarks.
    b. angiography.
    c. real-time ultrasound.
    d. radiography.

14. At the time of insertion of an NTHC into the femoral vein, what type of barrier precaution is advised for the patient?
    a. Head-to-toe sterile draping.
    b. Face mask.
    c. Standard access site sterile draping.
    d. Standard access site sterile draping and face mask.

15. The patient's NTHC should be replaced with a tunneled catheter if access for dialysis is needed for more than
    a. 24 hours.
    b. 48 hours.
    c. 5 days.
    d. 7 days.

16. The treatment that has been shown to provide the best overall benefit for patients such as Mr. Brock with acute kidney injury is
    a. furosemide
    b. IV normal saline.
    c. fenoldopam.
    d. nifedipine.

17. Mr. Brock rings the bell frequently and often complains about staff members, insisting that they are neglectful and incompetent. The best response is,
    a. "I'm so sorry you experienced that. What can I do to help you?"
    b. "I'm sure that the other staff members are doing their best."
    c. "There are many other patients who need help too."
    d. "That is terrible. They should provide better care."

18. The patient is diagnosed with acute tubular necrosis and becomes increasingly depressed and withdrawn, stating that he wants to die rather than continue to suffer and to face the prospect of ongoing hemodialysis. The most appropriate response is to
    a. reassure the patient that his condition will improve.
    b. remind the patient that he is young and has much to live for.
    c. provide the patient information about living with hemodialysis.
    d. ask the physician for a psychiatric referral.

19. Mr. Brock has entered the oliguric phase of acute tubular necrosis when urinary output falls to
    a. <200 mL/day.
    b. <300 mL/day.
    c. <400 mL/day.
    d. <500 mL/day.

20. Mr. Brock becomes increasingly restless, irritable, and anxious, and has nausea, muscle cramps, and numbness and tingling of the fingertips and around the mouth. The ECG shows irregularities. The most likely cause is
    a. hypokalemia
    b. hyperkalemia.
    c. hyponatremia.
    d. hypernatremia.

Section Description: Independent Questions, Group 1 (Questions 21 -32)

21. If a patient has allergic reactions during hemodialysis despite the use of a variety of different dialyzers and different dialysate solutions, the next steps should probably be to
    a. change to peritoneal dialysis.
    b. administer corticosteroids during hemodialysis.
    c. try heparin-free dialysis.
    d. use low-molecular-weight heparin.

22. Patients receiving hemodialysis should be advised to wash the access site before coming for treatment with
    a. isopropyl alcohol 70%.
    b. povidone iodine.
    c. chlorhexidine gluconate 2%.
    d. soap and water.

23. The purpose of a break tank or reduced pressure zone valve in the water system is to
    a. ensure adequate water supply.
    b. sterilize the water supply.
    c. decrease water pressure.
    d. prevent backflow.

24. When drawing a postdialysis blood sample for BUN, one method is to slow the blood flow rate to
    a. 200 mL/ min for 30 seconds.
    b. 100 mL/min for 15 seconds.
    c. 100 mL/min for 3 minutes.
    d. 200 mL/min for 3 minutes.

25. For short-term central venous catheters (CVCs) in adults, the CDC recommends that transparent dressings be changed at least every
    a. 24 hours.
    b. 2 days.
    c. 5 days.
    d. 7 days.

26. The external surface of the hemodialysis machine should be cleaned and disinfected at least
    a. every 8 hours.
    b. every 24 hours.
    c. after every patient.
    d. after every 2 patients.

27. When a patient is using home hemodialysis, the purpose of teaching the patient to "snap and tap" the tubing and filter is to
    a. remove air bubbles.
    b. straighten the tubing.
    c. prime the tubing with saline.
    d. improve patency.

28. Heparin should generally be administered during hemodialysis to maintain an ACT level of baseline plus
    a. 20%.
    b. 40%.
    c. 60%.
    d. 80%.

29. If routine heparin is administered for anticoagulation for hemodialysis with an initial bolus and subsequent infusion, the correct administration is
    a. inject bolus into arterial line, flush with saline, and then infuse heparin into venous line.
    b. inject bolus into venous line, flush with saline, and then infuse heparin into arterial line.
    c. inject bolus into venous line, flush with saline, and then infuse heparin into venous line
    d. inject bolus into arterial line, flush with saline, and then infuse heparin into arterial line.

30. After the initial heparin bolus for hemodialysis, when should dialysis be initiated?
    a. Immediately.
    b. 1 to 2 minutes.
    c. 3 to 5 minutes.
    d. 5 to 8 minutes.

31. According to the KDOQI guidelines, the minimum target spKt/V dose for patients receiving hemodialysis is
   a. 0.8.
   b. 1.
   c. 1.2.
   d. 1.4.

32. If a hemodialysis patient has a dialyzer clearance rate of 250 mL/min with 4-hour treatment, the total volume of blood cleared is
   a. 6 L.
   b. 60 L.
   c. 600 mL
   d. 600 L.

Section Description: Jackson Case Questions (Questions 33-43)

Kiante Jackson, a 38-year-old man with diabetes, has been diagnosed with chronic kidney disease.

33. When instructing a patient about collecting urine for a 24-hour creatinine clearance test, the patient should be advised to
   a. Begin saving urine with the first urination in the morning, and mark this as the beginning saving period.
   b. Discard the first urination in the morning and mark this as the beginning saving period.
   c. Begin saving urine with the first urination in the morning, but discard the first morning urination on the second day and end collection.
   d. Begin saving urine with the second urination in the morning and count that time as the beginning of the saving period.

34. If a patient is diagnosed with chronic kidney disease, the initial imaging is usually a(n)
   a. CT scan.
   b. MRI.
   c. X-ray.
   d. ultrasound.

35. Which medication(s) is recommended to control hypertension and slow the rate of chronic kidney disease in patients with diabetes mellitus?
   a. Beta-blocker.
   b. Calcium channel blocker.
   c. Loop diuretic.
   d. ACE inhibitor and ARB.

36. The KDIGO lipid guidelines recommend treatment with a statin or statin/ezetimibe combination for
   a. all patients with chronic kidney disease.
   b. all patient ≤50 years of age at stage 1 or 2 of chronic kidney disease.
   c. all patients ≥50 years of age with eGFR <60 mL/min/1.73 m² and not on dialysis.
   d. all patients at stage 5 kidney failure on dialysis.

37. Before therapy with an erythropoiesis-stimulating agent (ESA) is initiated with chronic kidney disease, which of the following should be assessed?
    a. GFR.
    b. BUN.
    c. Serum creatinine.
    d. Iron status.

38. Which of the following tests assesses the bioavailability of iron?
    a. Transferrin saturation = (serum iron level X 100)/total iron binding capacity.
    b. Serum ferritin.
    c. Serum iron binding capacity.
    d. Serum albumin.

39. If a nondialytic patient with chronic kidney disease requires treatment for iron deficiency anemia, KDIGO recommends as initial therapy
    a. IV low-molecular-weight iron.
    b. oral iron supplements.
    c. IV high-molecular-weight iron.
    d. increased dietary iron.

40. Kidney is generally considered inevitable when loss of kidney function reaches
    a. 30% to 40%.
    b. 40% to failure 50%.
    c. 50% to 60%.
    d. 60% to 70%.

41. If a high-pressure alarm for arterial pressure (pre-pump) sounds during hemodialysis, this could indicate
    a. vasoconstriction.
    b. drop in speed of blood pump.
    c. kink in arterial bloodline.
    d. infiltration of arterial needle.

42. A 40-year-old patient with chronic kidney disease and renal failure states he is concerned that the illness will affect his marriage and relationship with his spouse. What initial topic should the nurse likely discuss with the patient?
    a. Depression.
    b. Sexual dysfunction.
    c. Marriage counseling.
    d. Family issues.

43. The cardiac abnormality that is most prevalent in patients with chronic kidney disease and renal failure is
    a. right atrial hypertrophy.
    b. left atrial hypertrophy.
    c. left ventricular hypertrophy.
    d. right ventricular hypertrophy.

Section Description: Novak Case Questions (Questions 44-50)

Sarah Novak is a 35-year-old woman who had a kidney transplant because of adult-onset polycystic kidney disease, but the kidney transplant failed so she is again receiving hemodialysis while awaiting another kidney. Ms. Novak tends to develop hypotension during hemodialysis treatments.

44. Which of the following interventions may be indicated for a patient who develops hypotension during hemodialysis?
    a. Increasing the ultrafiltration rate near the end of the session.
    b. Administering hypotonic sodium solution IV.
    c. Utilizing sodium modeling.
    d. Administering midodrine (Orvaten).

45. If Ms. Novak has a blood flow rate of 400 and the serum urea nitrogen is 100 at inflow and 35 at outflow, the urea reduction ration (URR) expressed in percentages is
    a. 35%.
    b. 70%.
    c. 50%.
    d. 65%.

46. The nurse has calculated the target weight loss for Ms. Novak's hemodialysis session, but the patient insists that the nurse has made an error and that the target is 1 kg too high. The nurse should
    a. recalculate the target weight loss.
    b. ignore the patient.
    c. reassure the patient that the target is correct.
    d. advise the patient that 1 kg is inconsequential.

47. Weight gain between hemodialysis treatments should not exceed
    a. 1% of dry weight.
    b. 5% of dry weight.
    c. 8% of dry weight.
    d. 10% of dry weight.

48. Ms. Novak has a number of routine blood tests, including serum ferritin. The target for serum ferritin for patients on hemodialysis is
    a. ≥100 ng/mL.
    b. ≤100 ng/mL.
    c. ≥200 ng/mL.
    d. ≤200 ng/mL.

49. Ms. Novak insists on sipping water to relieve thirst during hemodialysis. How should fluid drunk during hemodialysis be accounted for?
    a. Fluid drunk during hemodialysis can be ignored.
    b. The total volume must be added to the total volume of fluid that must be removed.
    c. The total volume is accounted for in the next hemodialysis treatment.
    d. Half the volume should be added to the total fluid that must be removed.

50. Ms. Novak asks the nurse what the chance is that the disease will pass to any children if her spouse is disease free. The nurse should advise the patient that a child will
   a. have no risk of developing the disease.
   b. have a 25% risk of developing the disease.
   c. have a 50% risk of developing the disease.
   d. have a 100% risk of developing the disease.

Section Description: Rodriguez Case Questions (Questions 51-56)

> Raul Rodriguez is a 52-year-old man with diabetes and end-stage kidney disease. Mr. Rodriguez uses CAPD but reports that his peritoneal fluid has become cloudy.

51. Which of the following medications may result in cloudy peritoneal fluid for patients on peritoneal dialysis?
   a. Calcium carbonate.
   b. Beta-blockers.
   c. ACE inhibitors.
   d. Calcium channel blockers.

52. Which of the following places a patient with peritoneal dialysis at high risk for peritonitis?
   a. Spiking of dialysis bags.
   b. "Flush before fill" procedure.
   c. Double-cuffed catheter.
   d. Downward directed skin exit site.

53. Mr. Rodriguez's peritoneal catheter cultures positive for fungal organisms, indicating that the tube is colonized. The most likely intervention is
   a. antifungal instillations.
   b. removal of catheter and temporary hemodialysis.
   c. replacement of catheter.
   d. oral nystatin until culture is clear.

54. When patients are undergoing peritoneal dialysis, the most common pathway of infection resulting in peritonitis is
   a. periluminal.
   b. hematogenous.
   c. intraluminal.
   d. transvaginal.

55. If Mr. Rodriguez's CAPD requires a sample of peritoneal solution for evaluation of the cell count, the correct method of obtaining the specimen is to
   a. aspirate directly from the peritoneal catheter.
   b. invert the drainage bag a few times to mix the solution and aspirate from the bag port.
   c. aspirate from the bag port without mixing the solution.
   d. infuse 1 L of solution and then drain immediately and obtain sample from effluent.

56. If a sample of peritoneal fluid cannot be immediately processed, the inoculated culture bottles should ideally be stored at
    a. 35 °C.
    b. 35.5 °C.
    c. 37 °C.
    d. 38 °C.

Section Description: Independent Questions, Group 2 (Questions 57-73)

57. The most important factor in preventing exsanguination from dialysis line separation is
    a. functioning venous alarms.
    b. access site visibility.
    c. use of HemaClips.
    d. patient education.

58. The 3 bloodborne pathogens that pose the most risk for hemodialysis patients are
    a. hepatitis A, hepatitis B, and hepatitis C.
    b. hepatitis B, hepatitis C, and HIV.
    c. hepatitis B, Ebola, and HIV.
    d. hepatitis B, hepatitis D, and HIV.

59. A patient has pain and tightness in the chest with pain radiating to the jaw and down the left arm during hemodialysis. Before notifying the MD, the nurse's immediate intervention should be to
    a. slow the blood flow rate to 150 mL/min and decrease the ultrafiltration rate.
    b. increase the blood flow rate and the ultrafiltration rate by 20%.
    c. clamp all lines and stop dialysis.
    d. continue treatment without alteration.

60. The potassium level in dialysate is commonly
    a. 4 mM.
    b. 3 mM.
    c. 2 mM.
    d. 1 mM.

61. The first step in the Continuous Quality Improvement (CQI) process is to
    a. identify the need for improvement.
    b. analyze the process.
    c. identify root causes.
    d. implement plan-do-check-act (PDCA).

62. The 2 hormones produced by the kidneys are erythropoietin and
    a. calcitriol.
    b. calcium
    c. aldosterone.
    d. gastrin.

63. When instructing a patient on hemodialysis about weight gain, the patient should be advised that the usual goal for interdialytic weight gain is
    a. <0.5 kg/d.
    b. <1 kg/d.
    c. <1.5 kg/d.
    d. <2 kg/d.

64. If a patient has itching and stuffy nose that usually occurs only during hemodialysis, the most likely cause is
    a. hypersensitivity reaction.
    b. hepatitis.
    c. scabies.
    d. anxiety.

65. An elderly patient undergoing hemodialysis has expressed the wish to die but has never requested a DNR order. During treatment, the patient experiences a cardiac arrest. The correct initial response is to
    a. allow the patient to die.
    b. carry out CPR and defibrillation.
    c. carry out CPR only.
    d. call physician for guidance.

66. During hemodialysis, a patient who is lying in supine position has chest pain, begins coughing, and shows evidence of cyanosis of distal extremities and lips. The nurse suspects that the patient has
    a. anaphylaxis.
    b. myocardial infarction.
    c. disequilibrium symptom.
    d. air embolism.

67. Marked eosinophilia in a patient undergoing hemodialysis puts the patient at increased risk of
    a. type A (anaphylactic) dialyzer reaction.
    b. type B (hypersensitivity) dialyzer reaction.
    c. hemolysis.
    d. air embolism.

68. If severe hemolysis occurs during hemodialysis, for which electrolyte imbalance is the patient most at risk?
    a. Hyponatremia.
    b. Hypernatremia.
    c. Hypokalemia.
    d. Hyperkalemia.

69. The hemodialysis center has instituted a "zero lift" policy. The primary purpose of such a policy is to
    a. promote patient independence.
    b. prevent injuries.
    c. reduce liability.
    d. reduce staffing.

70. The legal document that assigns a healthcare proxy to make decisions in the event that a person is unable to do so is a(n)
    a. advance directive.
    b. living will.
    c. durable power of attorney.
    d. DNR.

71. If the administration of a dialysis center bills for good and services that were not provided, it can be prosecuted under which of the following acts?
    a. Public Health Service Act.
    b. Snyder Act.
    c. Affordable Care Act.
    d. False Claims Act.

72. When utilizing the "Got Chart" method of contacting a physician by telephone regarding a hemodialysis patient, the first step is to ensure
    a. there are no standing orders that pertain to the situation.
    b. the nurse has checked physician preferences regarding contact.
    c. the nurse has read the most recent progress notes.
    d. the nurse is contacting the correct physician.

73. When utilizing Maslow's Hierarchy of Needs to set priorities in nursing care for hemodialysis patients, which level of needs has the highest priority?
    a. Safety and security
    b. Love and belonging
    c. Self-esteem
    d. Physiologic

Section Description: Mason Case Questions (Questions 74-82)

Stanley Mason is a 68-year-old man with end-stage kidney disease. He has decided against a kidney transplant and will begin hemodialysis.

74. Mr. Mason is scheduled for "vessel mapping." The purpose of "vessel mapping," is to ensure
    a. the surgeon has completed the AV fistula properly.
    b. the blood flow distal to the AV fistula is adequate.
    c. the blood flow proximal to the AV fistula is adequate.
    d. the surgeon will find adequate vessels for the AV fistula.

75. Mr. Mason has a subsequent surgery to create an AV fistula. When determining if a new AV fistula is maturing, the three factors to palpate and assess are the
    a. pulse, sensitivity, and vessel growth.
    b. incision, pulse, and vessel growth.
    c. thrill, vessel growth, and vessel firmness.
    d. incision, vessel growth, and pulse.

76. Mr. Mason must decide what schedule of dialysis he wants. The dialysis center offers nighttime hemodialysis with 7- to 8-hour sessions 3 times weekly. Compared with the usual daytime schedule, the nighttime schedule
   a. offers no advantage.
   b. results in more complications.
   c. results in better survival rates.
   d. results in more food and fluid restrictions.

77. When Mr. Mason begins hemodialysis treatments, he brings food with him to eat during his hemodialysis treatment. Patients should be advised to avoid eating during hemodialysis because ingestion of food may result in
   a. hypotension.
   b. hypertension.
   c. nausea and vomiting.
   d. shivering and chills.

78. During treatment, the nurse takes care to place the needles in antegrade position. The most important reason for placing hemodialysis needles in antegrade position is because
   a. it is easier to place the needles in this manner.
   b. it is less painful for the patients.
   c. it causes less scarring.
   d. it decreases the chance of infection.

79. Mr. Mason has weakness, and the nurse notes increasing muscle atrophy of the legs, decreased range of motion, and difficulty walking. The nurse should
   a. advise the patient to be more active.
   b. advise the patient to utilize a walker to prevent falls.
   c. ask the patient to keep a record of activities.
   d. ask the physician to refer the patient for physical therapy.

80. Mr. Mason persists in smoking despite attempts to educate him about the risks of smoking. The patient points out that his parents and family members smoke, and all are relatively healthy. The nurse should advise the patient that
   a. risks of smoking are essentially the same for dialysis patients as for people without kidney disease.
   b. nicotine levels after smoking are higher in dialysis patients than in people without kidney diseases.
   c. the patient is at much greater risk from smoking than his family members.
   d. the patient should not compare himself with healthy family members.

81. Mr. Mason has chronic itching and wants to try herbal or complementary treatment, as medications have provided little relief. If a hemodialysis patient wants to try herbal or complementary medicine to control chronic itching, the therapy that may be most beneficial is
   a. acupuncture.
   b. aromatherapy.
   c. St. John's wort.
   d. therapeutic touch.

82. Five minutes after initiation of a hemodialysis treatment, the patient experiences of dyspnea, generalized itching, tingling about the mouth, and feeling faint. The patient has periorbital edema, and hives are evident. The nurse should immediately call for help and
   a. decrease the blood flow rate.
   b. increase the ultrafiltration rate.
   c. provide oxygen.
   d. clamp all lines and stop dialysis.

Section Description: Walker Case Questions (Questions 83-90)

> *MaryBeth Walker is a 28-year-old woman with a history of chronic glomerulonephritis affecting both kidneys. Because she is nearing end-stage kidney disease, she has decided to have hemodialysis treatments.*

83. Ideally, for a patient with chronic kidney disease who will eventually have to have hemodialysis, a phlebotomist should draw blood from the
   a. right antecubital area.
   b. left antecubital area.
   c. hand veins.
   d. foot veins.

84. How many months prior to the expected onset of dialysis should a patient such as Ms. Walker have an AV fistula created?
   a. 1 to 2 months.
   b. 2 to 4 months.
   c. 4 to 6 months.
   d. 6 to 9 months.

85. Dialysis is usually started in a patient with chronic kidney disease when the patient's eGFR falls to about
   a. 5 mL/min/1.73 m^2.
   b. 6.5. mL/min/1.73 m^2.
   c. 8 mL/min/1.73 m^2.
   d. 12 mL/min/1.73 m^2.

86. If Ms. Walker's PTH level is high, the most appropriate referral is likely to a(n)
   a. internist.
   b. nephrologist.
   c. endocrinologist.
   d. hematologist.

87. Ms. Walker should avoid MRI with gadolinium contrast agent because it may result in
   a. anaphylaxis.
   b. nephrogenic systemic fibrosis.
   c. glomerulonephritis.
   d. renal vascular stenosis.

88. When teaching Ms. Walker about dietary restrictions, the patient should be advised to limit dietary phosphorus intake to
   a. 400 to 600 mg/d.
   b. 600 to 800 mg/d.
   c. 800 to 1000 mg/d.
   d. 1000 to 1200 mg/d.

89. According to KDOQI guidelines, patients with chronic kidney disease should restrict calcium intake to
   a. 1200 mg/d.
   b. 1500 mg/d.
   c. 1800 mg/d.
   d. 2000 mg/d.

90. In a patient with chronic kidney disease, such as Ms. Walker, metabolic acidosis results in
   a. increased risk of cardiovascular disease.
   b. increased reabsorption of bone.
   c. increased risk of hemorrhage.
   d. increased risk of vascular calcification.

Section Description: Stanton Case Questions (Questions 91-94)

James Stanton is a 52-year-old man who has undergone a kidney transplantation.

91. Mr. Stanton is taking cyclosporine as an antirejection drug after kidney transplant, but he states that his general practitioner is concerned about his cholesterol level and has ordered atorvastatin. The nurse should
   a. call the physician to discuss possible adverse interactions.
   b. discuss side effects of atorvastatin with the patient.
   c. advise the patient not to take atorvastatin.
   d. tell the patient to take atorvastatin with food.

92. Because of immunosuppression, Mr. Stanton is at increased risk of infection. Following kidney transplantation and initiation of immunosuppression, the viral infection that is usually the most cause for concern is
   a. CMV.
   b. BKV.
   c. HCV.
   d. RSV.

93. According to the usual timeline of infections following kidney transplantation, when would infection a MRSA infection most likely develop?
   a. Within less than a month.
   b. Within 1 to 6 months.
   c. After 6 months.
   d. After 12 months.

94. Following the kidney transplantation, Mr. Stanton adheres closely to treatment regimens for the first 10 months and then begins missing physician appointments and failing to take all of prescribed medications, stating that he is doing fine and does not need to follow such a strict regimen. The defense mechanism the patient is using is
    a. repression.
    b. regression.
    c. denial.
    d. rationalization.

Section Description: Independent Questions, Group 3 (Questions 95 -115)

95. When considering the chain of infection, the 3 most common reservoirs of interest include humans, environment, and
    a. vectors.
    b. water.
    c. air.
    d. animals.

96. Which of the following immunoglobulins is the most prevalent and helps to protect the body against both viral and bacterial infections?
    a. IgA.
    b. IgM.
    c. IgE.
    d. IgG.

97. The primary reason that some hospital units ban fresh flowers and plants is because
    a. there is no room for them.
    b. they require too much time to care for.
    c. they may carry pathogenic organisms.
    d. they increase risk of injury from broken glass.

98. If 4 patients on a hospital unit develop infections with *Clostridium difficile* in 1 week, this would be classified as a(n)
    a. outbreak.
    b. cluster.
    c. epidemic.
    d. pandemic.

99. When an increase in infections occurs in a hospital unit, besides notifying the administration, which hospital unit should also be notified?
    a. Microbiology laboratory.
    b. Admissions.
    c. Pharmacy.
    d. Radiology.

100. If there is an outbreak of *Aspergillus* infections in patients hospitalized with chronic kidney disease, an outbreak investigation should include review of
   a. housekeeping procedures.
   b. handwashing procedures.
   c. the water system.
   d. construction projects.

101. The number one cause of kidney failure in the United States is
   a. polycystic kidney disease.
   b. hypertension.
   c. diabetes mellitus, type 2.
   d. heart failure.

102. A patient who cannot tolerate contrast for a CT is scheduled for an MRI to evaluate a mass on his kidney, but the nurse notes that the patient seems very nervous and upset as the time for the MRI approaches. On questioning, the patient confesses to the nurse that, although he understands the need for the MRI, he is very claustrophobic and worried about the procedure. The best solution is to
   a. reassure the patient that the MRI procedure is benign.
   b. advise the patient to close his eyes and practice relaxation during the MRI.
   c. contact the physician and request an order for a sedative.
   d. cancel the MRI.

103. Which of the following factors may produce a false negative finding in a urine dipstick for protein?
   a. Specific gravity of <1.01.
   b. Specific gravity of >1.03.
   c. Alkaline urine.
   d. Presence of blood.

104. Which of the following may result in ischemic injury to the kidneys rather than nephrotoxic injury?
   a. Radiopaque contrast dye.
   b. Amphetamines.
   c. Anaphylaxis.
   d. Tumor lysis syndrome.

105. According to the Renal Physicians Association's clinical practice guidelines to determine if dialysis should be avoided or stopped in patients with ESKD, one requirement is
   a. family consensus.
   b. malignant disease.
   c. life expectancy <1 year.
   d. shared decision making.

106. Which of the following is an example of a post-renal cause of acute kidney injury?
   a. Rhabdomyolysis.
   b. Prostatic hypertrophy.
   c. Acute glomerulonephritis.
   d. Sepsis.

107. Sepsis that is associated with renal ischemia may result in
    a. acute tubular necrosis.
    b. hydronephrosis.
    c. malignant hypertension.
    d. thrombosis.

108. A patient with chronic kidney disease has anorexia but is steadily increasing weight. The patient's potassium is 6.4 mEq/L, BUN 43 mg/dL, creatinine 3.6 mg/dL, hemoglobin 6.4 g/dL, and hematocrit 18.8%. Which of these laboratory findings has priority for intervention?
    a. Potassium.
    b. Creatinine.
    c. Hemoglobin.
    d. BUN.

109. A patient takes calcium carbonate 500 mg orally twice daily. Other medications include nifedipine extended-release (ER) 60 mg twice daily, aluminum hydroxide 600 mg three times daily, epoetin alfa 5000 units subcutaneously 3 times weekly, and iron polysaccharide complex 1 tablet daily. Which of these medications should not be taken at the same time as calcium carbonate?
    a. Nifedipine ER.
    b. Aluminum carbonate.
    c. Epoetin alfa.
    d. Iron polysaccharide complex.

110. Which of the patient's medications may increase risk of osteomalacia and refractory anemia?
    a. Nifedipine ER.
    b. Aluminum hydroxide.
    c. Epoetin alfa.
    d. Iron polysaccharide complex.

111. A patient with chronic kidney disease on dialysis has been prescribed cinacalcet (Sensipar), probably indicating that the patient has
    a. decreased parathyroid hormone.
    b. hyperkalemia.
    c. elevated parathyroid hormone.
    d. hypocalcemia.

112. When percussing the right kidney area of a patient using indirect fist percussion, the patient experiences pain when the nurse delivers a firm blow. This likely indicates
    a. normal finding.
    b. renal cell cancer.
    c. congenital malformation of the kidney.
    d. infection or polycystic kidney disease.

113. If a 24-hour urine quantitative protein test shows persistent proteinuria, this usually indicates
   a. congenital abnormality.
   b. kidney infection.
   c. renal tumor.
   d. glomerular renal disease.

114. Following a renal biopsy, a compression bandage should be applied to the needle insertion site and the patient positioned
   a. supine and at bedrest for 24 hours.
   b. on biopsy side for up to 60 minutes and bedrest for 24 hours.
   c. with no positional restrictions.
   d. on biopsy side for 4 hours and bedrest for 24 hours.

115. With the autosomal recessive form of medullary cystic disease, kidney failure usually occurs
   a. in infancy.
   b. before age 20.
   c. after age 20.
   d. between ages 30 and 40.

Section Description: Santos Case Questions (Questions 116-118)

Following treatment for leukemia, Maria Santos, a 50-year-old woman, develops tumor lysis syndrome.

116. Which of the following responses to cell lysis may result in urinary obstruction and decreased glomerular filtration rates, leading to renal insufficiency and acute kidney failure?
   a. Hypermagnesemia.
   b. Hypophosphatemia.
   c. Hyperuricemia.
   d. Hypercalcemia.

117. Which electrolyte imbalances are likely to occur with tumor lysis syndrome?
   a. Hyperkalemia, hyperphosphatemia, and hypocalcemia.
   b. Hypokalemia, hypophosphatemia, and hypercalcemia.
   c. Hyperkalemia, hypophosphatemia, and hypocalcemia.
   d. Hyperkalemia, hyperphosphatemia, and hypercalcemia.

118. If Ms. Santos requires treatment for hyperuricemia, which of the following medications may be utilized to prevent uric acid crystallization?
   a. Loop diuretic.
   b. Thiazide diuretic.
   c. Alkalinizing agent.
   d. Uricosuric agent.

Section Description: Chan Case Questions (Questions 119-125)

Joe Chan, a 63-year-old man, has stage 4 chronic kidney disease and is considering options for when his disease worsens.

119. When discussing disease progression with a patient such as Mr. Chan with chronic kidney disease, kidney transplantation should be initially considered
    a. if patients have repeated access failure.
    b. after a trial period of dialysis.
    c. at stage 4 of chronic kidney disease.
    d. at stage 5 of chronic kidney disease.

120. As Mr. Chan nears end-stage kidney disease, he decides that he wants to be put on the list for a kidney transplant. Mr. Chan is evaluated by a psychiatrist with the Mini-Mental State Examination to determine if he is a good candidate for transplantation. Which of the following scores is within normal range?
    a. ≥10.
    b. ≥15.
    c. ≥24.
    d. ≥40.

121. A casual acquaintance of Mr. Chan has volunteered to donate a kidney to him. When considering whether a potential unrelated kidney donor is acceptable, which of the following should raise concerns?
    a. The potential donor has made repeated reports about donating on multiple social media sites.
    b. The potential donor asks many questions about what to expect in the postoperative period.
    c. The potential donor is independently wealthy and is not employed.
    d. The potential donor reports transient episode of depression as an adolescent.

122. Mr. Chan subsequently receives a kidney transplant. Following the kidney transplant, Mr. Chan becomes agitated and confused with periods of lucidity, typical of delirium. The initial response should be
    a. reorientation and comfort measures.
    b. haloperidol.
    c. restraints and sitters.
    d. quetiapine.

123. While receiving renal transplant medications, Mr. Chan has been experiencing visual hallucinations. Which of the following medications is most likely the cause?
    a. Prednisone.
    b. Lamivudine.
    c. Tacrolimus.
    d. Cyclosporine.

124. What dietary restrictions are common for patients on cyclosporine as renal transplant medication?
   a. Patients should avoid dairy products within 2 hours of medication.
   b. Patients should avoid grapefruit and foods high in potassium.
   c. Patients should avoid foods high in magnesium.
   d. Patients should avoid red meat and high protein foods.

125. For the immediate postoperative period following kidney transplantation, patients should be advised to have daily protein intake of
   a. 0.8 g/kg/d.
   b. 0.8 to 1 g/kg/d.
   c. 1 to 1.2 g/kg/d.
   d. 1.3 to 1.5 g/kg/d.

Section Description: Stein Case Questions (Questions 126-128)

Rachel Stein is an 80-year-old woman with stage 3 chronic kidney disease.

126. When assessing an 80-year-old patient for kidney function, the nurse expects age-related changes to result in
   a. decreased kidney size, decreased creatinine clearance, and increased BUN and serum creatinine.
   b. increased kidney size, increased creatinine clearance, and decreased BUN and serum creatinine.
   c. decreased kidney size, decreased creatinine clearance, BUN, and serum creatinine.
   d. decreased kidney size, increased creatinine clearance, and increased BUN and serum creatinine.

127. Stage 3 chronic kidney disease is characterized by
   a. eGFR 15 to 29 mL/min.
   b. eGFR 30 to 59 mL/min.
   c. eGFR 60 to 89 mL/min.
   d. eGFR ≥90 mL/min.

128. For elderly patients with chronic kidney disease who do not exhibit marked fluid overload, the need for dialysis may be delayed up to 1 year with
   a. protein restriction and ketoacids.
   b. fluid and protein restrictions.
   c. protein restrictions and loop diuretics.
   d. fluid restriction and ketoacids.

Section Description: Woods Case Questions (Questions 129-135)

James Woods is a 68-year old man with end-stage kidney disease. He has been maintained on hemodialysis but has had to have repeated surgical procedures for vascular access and now wants to have a kidney transplant.

129. Mr. Woods is a candidate for kidney transplantation. The patient must register with the
     a. American Organization Transplant Association (AOTA).
     b. Organ Procurement and Transplantation Network (OPTN).
     c. United Network for Organ Sharing (UNOS).
     d. American Transplant Foundation (ATF).

130. When a patient such as Mr. Woods is on the waiting list for a kidney transplantation, what 3 factors are evaluated to determine if a match is appropriate?
     a. blood type, HLA factors, and ages of donor and recipient
     b. blood type, HLA factors, and race
     c. blood type, HLA factors, and antigens
     d. blood type, HLA factors, and antibodies

131. If Mr. Woods expresses concern that his insurance and available resources will not cover all of the cost of kidney transplantation, what Internet resource may provide the most valuable information?
     a. CMS (Medicare/Medicaid).
     b. UNOS Transplant Living.
     c. National Kidney Foundation.
     d. National Cancer Institute.

132. Because Mr. Woods is concerned about the lengthy wait for a kidney, he is willing to consider a marginal kidney or a dual kidney transplantation. Which of the following would classify a cadaveric kidney donor as a marginal or expanded criteria donor (ECD) according to UNOS criteria?
     a. Age 55 at death.
     b. Terminal creatinine of 1.3 mg/dL.
     c. Previous history of slight cardiovascular accident (CVA).
     d. Recent onset of hypertension.

133. The primary purpose of dual kidney transplantation is to
     a. provide more normal physiologic functioning.
     b. increase success rates of marginal kidneys.
     c. provide insurance in case one kidney fails.
     d. prevent recurrent glomerular disease.

134. Which of the following is one of the critical major histocompatibility complex (MHC) genes for matching donor and recipient?
     a. HLA-C.
     b. HLA-DQ.
     c. HLA-DP.
     d. HLA-DR.

135. Following kidney transplantation, patients have increased risk of malignancies. The most common cancer that develops after transplantation is
   a. renal cell carcinoma.
   b. lymphoma.
   c. skin cancer.
   d. liver cancer.

Section Description: Independent Questions, Group 4 (Questions 136 -150)

136. According to the RIFLE (**R**isk, **I**njury, **F**ailure, **L**oss, **E**nd-stage kidney disease) criteria, the stage of failure occurs with
   a. serum creatinine increased by 1.5 times.
   b. GFR increased by 25%.
   c. GFR decreased by 50%.
   d. urine output <0.3 mL/kg/h for 24 hours.

137. During the diuretic phase of acute kidney injury, the patient should be closely monitored for dehydration, hyponatremia, and
   a. hypokalemia.
   b. hypocalcemia.
   c. hypophosphatemia.
   d. hyperkalemia.

138. If a patient with acute kidney injury is prescribed sodium polystyrene sulfonate (Kayexalate), which of the following is a contraindication to administration of the drug?
   a. Diabetes mellitus.
   b. Controlled hypertension.
   c. Nausea.
   d. Paralytic ileus.

139. When considering the stages of chronic kidney disease, a patient is considered in need of dialysis when the GFR falls to
   a. 60 to 89 mL/min/1.73 m^2.
   b. 30 to 59 mL/min/1.73 m^2.
   c. <15 mL/min/1.73 m^2.
   d. <10 mL/min/1.73 m^2.

140. The primary treatment for chronic kidney disease-mineral and bone disorder (CKD-MBD) is decreasing
   a. hyperphosphatemia.
   b. hypercalcemia.
   c. hypernatremia.
   d. hyperkalemia.

141. Standards that cover medical devices used for dialysis, such as dialyzers and blood tubing, are set by
   a. ESRD Network.
   b. The Joint Commission.
   c. FDA.
   d. AAMI.

142. If a patient with uremia passes urine that is foamy or bubbly, this probably represents
   a. protein in the urine.
   b. rapid urination.
   c. phosphate crystals.
   d. normal urinary finding.

143. If imaging shows that the kidneys have atrophied to about one-fifth the normal size, the most likely diagnosis is
   a. acute glomerulonephritis.
   b. chronic glomerulonephritis.
   c. polycystic kidney disease.
   d. renal cell cancer.

144. Patients are at increased risk of mortality when predialytic albumin levels fall to
   a. <2 g/dL.
   b. <3 g/dL.
   c. <4 g/dL.
   d. <5 g/dL.

145. Treatment for nephrotic syndrome usually includes diuretics, lipid-lowering agents, and
   a. ACE inhibitors.
   b. beta-blockers.
   c. calcium channel blockers.
   d. vasodilators.

146. Which part of the nephron resorbs urea, glucose, and amino acids?
   a. Proximal convoluted tubule.
   b. Loop of Henle.
   c. Glomerulus.
   d. Bowman's capsule.

147. An 80-year-old patient fell at home, fracturing her right hip. She was unable to move and lay on the floor for 24 hours before rescue. Routine medications include a beta-blocker and statin. On admission to the hospital, the patient's urine is dark in color. The patient experiences generalized muscle weakness and pain. Laboratory tests indicate elevated creatine phosphokinase, serum myoglobin, and urinary myoglobin. Based on these findings, the patient is at risk of
   a. pulmonary embolism.
   b. stroke.
   c. rhabdomyolysis.
   d. fat embolism syndrome.

148. A 44-year-old man with a history of diabetes mellitus and hypertension is admitted to the hospital with increasing peripheral edema (2+ pitting), nausea and vomiting, lethargy, and generalized itching. The patient's BP is 190/120 mm Hg, pulse 86 bpm, respiration 26 breaths per minute. The patient's potassium (6.1 mmol/L) and phosphorus (10.2 mg/dL) were elevated and BUN was 150 mg/dL and serum creatinine 14 mg/dL. Parathyroid hormone level was 885 pg/mL. Hemoglobin was 8.4 g/dL and hematocrit 27.2%. Glucose is 106 mg/dL. Based on these findings, the patient is most likely experiencing
    a. liver failure.
    b. heart failure.
    c. rhabdomyolysis.
    d. uremia.

149. For most patients on CAPD, glucose present in the dialysate adds about how many calories each day?
    a. 200.
    b. 300.
    c. 500.
    d. 700.

150. The surface area of the peritoneal cavity in an adult is typically
    a. 0.5 to 1 m^2.
    b. 1 to 2 m^2.
    c. 2 to 3 m^2.
    d. 3 to 4 m^2.

Section Description: Davis Case Questions (Questions 151-153)

> *Maureen Davis is a 70-year-old woman with diabetes mellitus, hypertension, and end-stage-kidney disease. She is to have a catheter implanted for peritoneal dialysis and wants to try CAPD rather than hemodialysis.*

151. How long prior to a patient's beginning peritoneal dialysis should a catheter be implanted?
    a. 1 week.
    b. 2 weeks.
    c. 6 weeks.
    d. 2 months.

152. When teaching Ms. Davis about peritoneal dialysis, the nurse should advise the patient that one advantage to peritoneal dialysis over hemodialysis is
    a. fewer restrictions in fluids and sodium.
    b. fewer treatments needed.
    c. less potential for complications.
    d. lower restriction on phosphorus intake.

153. The nurse is concerned that Ms. Davis may not be a good candidate for CAPD. Which of the following is often a contraindication for peritoneal dialysis?
   a. Obesity.
   b. Young adulthood.
   c. Residual urinary function.
   d. Cardiovascular disease.

Section Description: Nguyen Case Questions (Questions 154-155)

Joy Nguyen is a 58-year-old woman with diabetes, type 2, and end-stage kidney disease. She has been treated with hemodialysis for 2 years.

154. Ms. Nguyen has developed numerous very painful firm brown nodules on both lower legs with some of the nodules eroding and become necrotic. The skin color appears mottled, and the patient has decreased sensation. The most likely cause of these symptoms is
   a. calcific uremic arteriolopathy (CUA).
   b. peripheral arterial disease (PAD).
   c. peripheral venous insufficiency.
   d. *Staphylococcus aureus* infection.

155. Based on these symptoms, the most likely intervention is
   a. corticosteroids.
   b. immunosuppressive agents.
   c. IV antibiotics.
   d. IV sodium thiosulfate.

Section Description: Bell Case Questions (Questions 156-159)

John Bell is a 48-year-old man who has been undergoing hemodialysis for 6 months.

156. Mr. Bell frequently experiences leg cramps during hemodialysis. Which of the following may result in muscle cramping during hemodialysis?
   a. Hypervolemia.
   b. Hypovolemia.
   c. Low ultrafiltration rate.
   d. High-sodium dialysis solution.

157. Mr. Bell says that he is unable to work or care for his family and is increasingly sedentary because of severe episodes of fatigue. The most important intervention is to
   a. advise a program of exercise.
   b. refer to a social worker.
   c. refer for psychological counseling.
   d. assess for causes of fatigue.

158. When documenting observations about a patient, which of the following is the most appropriate description?
   a. "Patient is nervous and upset."
   b. "Patient appears to be in a very good mood today."
   c. "Patient is sighing and rubbing hands together."
   d. "Patient is uncooperative and belligerent."

159. The patient has developed a small aneurysm and asks the nurse to cannulate the aneurysm for the hemodialysis treatment because another patient told Mr. Bell that it would be less painful than cannulation of the fistula. The best response is
   a. agree to cannulate the aneurysm.
   b. tell the patient that there is no reduced pain if cannulating the aneurysm.
   c. advise the patient that cannulating an aneurysm may result in rupture.
   d. tell the patient that the other patient was wrong.

Section Description: Independent Questions, Group 5 (Questions 160 -175)

160. The primary advantage of using a Y-set with preattached double-bag system rather than a straight set for peritoneal dialysis is
   a. ease of use.
   b. cost savings.
   c. decreased incidence of peritonitis.
   d. time saving.

161. A patient undergoing peritoneal dialysis and recovering from *Staphylococcus aureus* peritonitis is found to be a nasal carrier of *Staph*. The most commonly used prophylaxis is
   a. rifampin 300 mg daily for 1 month.
   b. rifampin 300 mg twice daily for 5 days every 4 weeks.
   c. mupirocin cream intranasally once daily indefinitely.
   d. mupirocin cream intranasally twice daily for 5 days every 4 weeks.

162. When teaching a patient about peritoneal dialysis and dwell times, the patient should understand that the minimum dwell time necessary for adequate removal of waste products is usually about
   a. 1 hour.
   b. 2 hours.
   c. 3 hours.
   d. 4 hours.

163. Which of the following is a risk factor for development of hernia in patients undergoing peritoneal dialysis?
   a. Small volumes of dialysate.
   b. Supine position during dwell.
   c. Anorexia and weight loss.
   d. Obesity.

164. If a patient has been experiencing recent weight gain without generalized edema but with protuberant abdomen, and if the returns of dialysate are less than the instilled volume, the nurse should suspect
    a. ultrafiltration failure.
    b. abdominal wall leak.
    c. overhydration.
    d. peritonitis.

165. Following insertion of a peritoneal catheter and beginning of peritoneal dialysis, the nurse notes that the dressing over the site is damp. Which of the following tests should be done to help determine if the cause is pericatheter leak?
    a. Protein dipstick.
    b. Glucose dipstick.
    c. Hemoglobin dipstick.
    d. Ketones dipstick.

166. If a patient tests positive for a pericatheter leak, the most common treatment is
    a. stopping peritoneal dialysis for up to 48 hours.
    b. surgical repairing of catheter site.
    c. removing peritoneal catheter and replacing at same site.
    d. removing peritoneal catheter and using an alternate site.

167. During the first dwell of peritoneal dialysis, a patient suddenly has severe shortness of breath. The immediate response should be to
    a. sit the patient upright.
    b. administer oxygen.
    c. stop the dialysis.
    d. advise the patient to take deep breaths and relax.

168. If a patient on CAPD has severe unremitting lower back pain, the best solution may be
    a. changing to APD with no daytime dwell.
    b. changing to APD with daytime dwell.
    c. a regimen of strengthening exercises for back and abdomen.
    d. remaining in supine position for an hour after completing a dwell.

169. Long-term peritoneal dialysis places the patient at increased risk for which electrolyte imbalance?
    a. Hyperkalemia.
    b. Hypokalemia.
    c. Hypocalcemia.
    d. Hypercalcemia.

170. The nurse serves as case manager for a patient who lives at considerable distance from the nurse's office in a rural area. The patient uses CAPD and manages fairly well but is anxious about being so far from medical help. The best method of keeping in touch with the patient and managing the patient's care is probably
    a. email.
    b. home visits.
    c. office visits.
    d. video chat.

171. A new occupational therapist has started working with the dialysis team, but this therapist has a different approach that the previous therapist, and some of the team members have begun complaining. As supervisor, the nurse's primary concern should be
    a. ensuring that the team members are satisfied and working together well.
    b. informing the occupational therapist about needed changes in approach.
    c. assessing the quality of care the occupational therapist provides.
    d. establishing authority over the occupational therapist.

172. When a patient is being discharged from the hospital and will be referred to a home health agency for assistance with peritoneal dialysis, the best method to ensure that the patient understands the discharge plan is to
    a. have the patient complete a post-discharge survey.
    b. telephone the patient after discharge to discuss the discharge plan.
    c. mail the patient a reminder of the discharge plan.
    d. ask the home health agency for a follow-up report.

173. If a hemodialysis patient routinely experiences hypotensive episodes near the end of a session, and malaise, muscle cramps, and dizziness after dialysis, what is the most likely cause?
    a. The dry weight is set too low.
    b. The dry weight is set too high.
    c. The patient is having an allergic reaction to dialysate.
    d. The patient is exhibiting signs of hypokalemia.

174. Patients undergoing home nocturnal hemodialysis are required to have which item within arm's reach while undergoing dialysis?
    a. Tourniquet.
    b. Kelly clamp.
    c. Whistle.
    d. Telephone.

175. For an end-stage kidney disease patient with difficulty sleeping because of restless legs syndrome, which of the following medications is generally considered the medication of choice?
    a. SSRI.
    b. Benzodiazepine.
    c. Dopamine precursor.
    d. Steroids.

Answers and Explanations

Section Description: Eggers Case Questions

1. B: If an 18-year-old patient using APD (also known as CCPD) has become increasingly withdrawn, answering in monosyllables and exhibiting a flat affect, the patient may benefit most from psychological counseling, as these are indications of depression. Depression is common with dialysis patients, especially adolescents, because of the many physical, social, and emotional demands of maintaining the dialysis schedule and coping with complications. The primary concern as the patient becomes more withdrawn is nonadherence with the treatment regimen.

2. A: If a patient is using APD with long day dwell, icodextrin could be used as the "last bag option." Many cyclers include the option to use a different dialysate for the last bag, which will be retained for an extended period of time. Icodextrin is only used for long dwells, so it is not appropriate for the nighttime cycles. Icodextrin induces ultrafiltration but is absorbed more slowly by the lymphatics than glucose solutions so there is no advantage to using it for short dwells.

3. C: If a patient has not been adhering to a healthy diet and the physician orders amino acid–based dialysate solution for nutritional supplementation, this solution should be used for one 4- to 6-hour dwell daily as the amino acids are absorbed during this period. If the amino acid dialysate solution (usually 1.1% essential and non-essential amino acids in a non-glucose solution) is used more than once daily, it may cause acidosis and increased serum urea.

4. D: Because the patient loses water-soluble vitamins during dialysis, these vitamins should be replaced with supplementation. Folate is especially lost, so patients should take vitamin B9 (folic acid is the synthetic form) as well as other B vitamins including vitamin B1 (thiamine), vitamin B2 (riboflavin), vitamin B3 (niacin), vitamin B7 (biotin), vitamin B5 (pantothenic acid), and vitamin B12 (cobalamins). Vitamins A, D, and K are fat-soluble vitamins. Vitamins A and K supplementation should be avoided.

5. A: If a patient on peritoneal dialysis receives calcium carbonate as a phosphate binder, 2 to 2.5 mEq/L of calcium is usually contained in the PD solution used for dialysis rather than 3.5 mEq/L, which was more commonly used with other phosphate binders. Lowering the concentration helps to prevent hypercalcemia that may result from oral intake of calcium and vitamin D. The lower calcium concentration may also help prevent adynamic bone disease, but it may result in higher levels of PTH.

6. A: When teaching a patient who is to undergo peritoneal dialysis about peritoneal transport and absorption of fluid per the lymphatics, the patient should understand that peritoneal fluid is usually absorbed at the rate of 1 to 2 mL/min. Absorption per the lymphatics is done at a fairly constant state with little variation, but absorption may be affected by various factors, including the intraperitoneal hydrostatic pressure and the overall efficiency of the lymphatics.

7. A: If a patient on peritoneal dialysis reports a break in sterile technique that may have resulted in contamination of the peritoneal cavity, the nurse expects that the immediate

response will be to institute preventive antimicrobial treatment; however, it is not clear that doing so will prevent peritonitis. A commonly used prophylaxis is ciprofloxacin. Additionally, the transfer set should be changed and the peritoneal cavity flushed with an antibiotic solution. Most organisms have incubation periods that range from 12 to 48 hours.

8. C: If the patient on peritoneal dialysis tests positive for peritonitis, the usually recommended method of administration for antibiotics is intraperitoneal unless the patient has evidence of systemic disease, and then the medication is administered intravenously. Patients are administered an intraperitoneal loading dose initially and thereafter antibiotics are added to each exchange or to one or more exchanges daily. The choice of antibiotic depends on the causative agent and whether or not the patient has residual urinary output.

9. A: Because of changes in permeability of the peritoneum resulting from peritonitis, the patient should be carefully monitored for hyperglycemia because of more rapid absorption of glucose. Diabetic patients are especially at risk. Serum glucose levels should be carefully monitored and insulin administration titrated as necessary. The increased permeability also results in more rapid absorption of fluid, which can result in fluid overload. Loss of protein may be increased during the episode of peritonitis.

10. C: Research regarding the use of prophylactic nystatin for patients receiving antibiotics for peritonitis and undergoing peritoneal dialysis is inconclusive. Fungal infections are often preceded by administration of antibiotics. However, if the rate of baseline fungal infections is high in a center, then prophylactic administration of nystatin may be indicated. Prophylaxis may prevent some *Candida* infections. Nystatin is usually administered orally throughout the course of antibiotics. The antibiotics are most often administered intraperitoneally.

11. A: If a patient undergoing peritoneal dialysis and being treated for peritonitis develops fibrinous clots in the peritoneal fluid (a common problem that occurs with peritonitis), the usual treatment is the addition of heparin to the dialysis solution. Usually 500 to 1000 units/L is added to the solution until the peritonitis no longer requires treatment and there is no evidence of fibrinous clots in the dialysis effluent. Fibrinous clots may result in blockage of the catheter.

Section Description: Brock Case Questions

12. D: Retroperitoneal hemorrhage is a serious complication of femoral catheterization. Other complications, common to all insertion sites, include hematoma, arterial puncture, and bloodstream infection. Bloodstream infection often causes the greatest risk. Both the use of the internal jugular vein and the subclavian vein increase risk of air embolus and pneumothorax. Central venous stenosis and arrhythmias may also occur. Femoral catheterization should be the site of last resort and should be avoided if other sites are accessible.

13. C: In order to reduce the risk of complications, when a non-tunneled temporary hemodialysis catheter (NTHC) is inserted into the femoral vein (or any other vein), the practitioner should use real-time ultrasound because vascular injuries, such as arterial punctures and hematomas, are fairly common if the practitioner uses only anatomic landmarks because of individual anatomic variation, especially in the position of the

femoral artery and the femoral vein. While uncommon (about 0.5%), femoral catheterization may result in severe hemorrhage, so correct catheter placement is critical.

14. A: At the time of insertion of a non-tunneled temporary hemodialysis catheter (NTHC) into the femoral vein (or any vein), the barrier precaution advised for the patient is head-to-toe sterile draping. A chlorhexidine scrub (2%) is recommended for antisepsis, using a back-and-forth method of cleansing and allowing the solution to dry on the skin according to manufacturer's recommendations. The healthcare provider should use maximal barrier protection, including gown, mask, cap, and gloves.

15. C: The patient's non-tunneled temporary hemodialysis catheter (NTHC) should be replaced with a tunneled catheter if access for dialysis is needed for more than 5 days because of the increased risk of bloodstream infections with non-tunneled catheters. NTHCs may be left in place for up to 7 days with access sites in the internal jugular and subclavian veins. NTHCs should not be placed if dialysis access is expected for a period of longer than 3 weeks.

16. B: The treatment that has been shown to provide the best overall benefit for patients with acute kidney injury is IV normal saline, administered to maintain a state of euvolemia or hypervolemia. Loop diuretics, such as furosemide, are frequently used to help maintain fluid balance but have not been shown to affect outcomes. Fenoldopam is sometimes used with hypertension to increase renal blood flow. Calcium channel blockers, such as nifedipine, are used as vasodilators/muscle relaxants, but their effectiveness is unclear.

17. A: If a patient with acute kidney injury receiving temporary hemodialysis rings the bell frequently and often complains about staff members, insisting that they are neglectful and incompetent, the best response is, "I'm so sorry you experienced that. What can I do to help?" It is important to acknowledge the patient's feelings without assigning blame to the patient or others and to attempt to alleviate the problem. Simply spending extra time with the patient may help to allay the patient's anxiety.

18. D: If a patient diagnosed with acute tubular necrosis becomes increasingly depressed and withdrawn, stating that he wants to die rather than continue to suffer and to face the prospect of ongoing hemodialysis, the most appropriate response is to ask the physician for a psychiatric referral for the patient. Because the patient may, in fact, require ongoing hemodialysis if the condition becomes chronic, it is important to remain truthful, but the patient may need professional intervention to assess his depression and suicidal ideation.

19. C: The patient has entered the oliguric phase of acute tubular necrosis when urinary output falls to <400 mL/day. The initial (onset) phase lasts for a few hours to a few days. It is followed in some patients by the oliguric or anuric phase, which lasts 10 to 16 days in oliguric patients. Some patients are nonoliguric; if this is the case, this phase lasts only 5 to 8 days. The third phase, the diuretic phase, lasts 7 to 14 days and includes a rise in GFR. The last stage is the recovery phase, which may take up to 2 years, although many patients never completely recover kidney function and about 5% require ongoing hemodialysis.

20. B: If the patient becomes increasingly restless, irritable, and anxious, and experiences nausea, muscle cramps, numbness and tingling of the fingertips and around the mouth, and ECG irregularities, the most likely cause is hyperkalemia, a common finding with acute tubular necrosis, especially during the oliguric phase. Metabolic acidosis may also occur.

The GFR decreases, resulting in increased BUN (azotemia), as well as hyperkalemia and other electrolyte imbalances, including hyperphosphatemia and hypocalcemia.

Section Description: Independent Questions, Group 1

21. C: If a patient has persistent allergic reactions during hemodialysis despite the use of a variety of different dialyzers and different dialysate solutions, the next steps should probably be to try heparin-free dialysis or citrate anticoagulation. Heparin may cause some patients to experience an allergic response, but low-molecular-weight heparin should not be used as a substitute because of cross-reactivity. If after a trial period of heparin-free dialysis the allergic reactions persist, then further investigation is warranted.

22. D: Patients receiving hemodialysis should be advised to wash the access site before coming for treatment with soap and water. Because *Staphylococcus aureus* may colonize at the access site, poor hygiene increases the risk of infection, so patients should be advised of the importance of good hygiene and should be trained to bathe regularly and wash the access site daily and before hemodialysis treatments. Patients should also be advised to monitor healthcare personnel to ensure they are using proper aseptic techniques and proper handwashing.

23. D: The purpose of a break tank or reduced pressure zone valve in the water system is to prevent backflow. If water pressure falls in the water distribution system, such as may occur with a line break or high water demand, water connected to the supply line from underground sources or storage tanks may backflow into the water system, resulting in contaminations. The break tank or reduced pressure zone valve prevents chemicals that have been removed during dialysis from entering the public water system and prevents contaminated water from entering the water distribution system.

24. B: When drawing a postdialysis blood sample for BUN, one method is to slow the blood flow rate to 100 mL/min for 15 seconds before sampling, as this duration of time is sufficient for unrecirculated blood to reach below the sampling port. As an alternative, the dialysate flow can be stopped for 3 minutes (or decreased to the minimum level if the equipment does not allow stopping the flow). This period of time is generally sufficient to stabilize the dialysate outlet BUN level with the blood inlet BUN level.

25. D: For short-term CVCs in adults, the CDC recommends that transparent dressings be changed every 7 days unless they become loosened and require more frequent changes. Gauze dressings should be changed every 2 days. Following the insertion of the CVC, the CDC recommends the initial dressing be changed only every 7 days until the exit site is well healed; more frequent dressing changes increase the risk of contamination of the exit site and infection.

26. C: The external surface of the hemodialysis machine should be cleansed and disinfected after every patient. If water or dialysate has sat in the hemodialysis machine overnight, then all of the fluid distribution system must be disinfected prior to the first utilization of the equipment for hemodialysis in the morning. Care must be taken to ensure that waste does not backflow into the machine. Most hemodialysis machines in the United States are single-pass machines in which all dialysate is discarded through a drain.

27. A: When a patient is utilizing home hemodialysis, the purpose of teaching the patient to "snap and tap" the tubing and filter is to remove air bubbles. Once the filter and tubing is attached to the equipment, it is primed with normal saline, and this clears out the air, but some bubbles may remain, and snapping and tapping helps to move the bubbles. Some microbubbles may persist, but large bubbles pose a risk and should be removed. The filter should be checked carefully for streaking, which can indicate an air pocket. The snap and tap procedure may take 5 to 15 minutes.

28. D: Heparin should generally be administered during hemodialysis to maintain an ACT level of baseline plus 80%. The level at the end of dialysis should be baseline plus 40%. If patients are at risk for bleeding and heparin-free dialysis resulted in clotting, then a tight heparin protocol is followed. With tight heparin, the ACT should be maintained at baseline plus 40% during dialysis and at the end of dialysis. The initial bolus dose is lower, 750 units, and the heparin infusion is initiated at the rate of 600 units per hour, but adjusted to maintain baseline plus 40%.

29. B: If routine heparin (unfractionated) is administered for anticoagulation for hemodialysis with an initial bolus (usually 2000 units) and subsequent infusion, the correct administration is to inject the bolus into venous line, flush with saline, and then infuse heparin (usually 1200 units per hour) into the arterial line. An alternative method for routine heparinization is to administer an initial higher bolus (such as 4000 units) and then give 1000 unit to 2000 unit boluses as need.

30. C: After the initial heparin bolus for hemodialysis, dialysis should be initiated in 3 to 5 minutes, which provides times for the heparin to disperse. Anticoagulation is important during dialysis because the blood must come in contact with a variety of different surfaces and membranes, all of which may result in the thrombus formation and blood clotting. Without anticoagulation, the thrombus formation may result in occlusion within the circuit.

31. D: According to the KDOQI guidelines, the minimum target spKt/V (single pool Kt/V) dose for patients receiving hemodialysis is 1.4 because the minimum dose for the patient is 1.2, but since there is a coefficient of variation among patients of 0.1 Kt/V units, the target dose is slightly higher to ensure the dose does not fall below 1.2. K refers to the dialyzer clearance of urea, t refers to the time/duration of dialysis, and V refers to the volume of body fluid (urea clearance area); the spKt/V is used to determine the adequacy of dialysis.

32. B: If a hemodialysis patient has a dialyzer clearance rate of 250 mL/min with a 4-hour treatment, the total volume of blood cleared is 60 L:
- 250 mL X 240 min = 60,000 mL or 60 L.

This clearance rate is used to calculate the Kt/V dose. The V refers to the total volume of fluid in the body, usually about 60% by weight; so if a patient weighs 70 kg, the volume of water in the body is 70 X .6 = 42 L.
- Kt = 250 X 240 = 60 L
- V = 70 X .6 = 42.
- Kt/V = 60/42 = 1.4

Section Description: Jackson Case Questions

33. B: When instructing a patient about collecting urine for a 24-hour creatinine clearance test, the patient should be advised to discard the first urination in the morning and mark

this as the beginning saving period. The 24-hour collection period should end after collecting the first urination in the morning of the second day. Normal values for creatinine clearance vary but are about 95 ± 20 mL/min for females and 125 ± 25 mL/min for males.

34. D: If a patient is diagnosed with chronic kidney disease, the initial imaging is usually an ultrasound because it uses sound waves to create images and is noninvasive, relatively inexpensive, and can show the size and position of the kidneys as well as any structural abnormalities and other abnormal findings, such as tumors or stones. X-rays may not show enough detail. Sometimes, the ultrasound is followed by a CT with contrast if indicated (such as when a tumor is found) or with an MRI.

35. D: The medications that are recommended to control hypertension and slow the rate of chronic kidney disease in patients with diabetes mellitus are ACE inhibitors and ARBs. This medication combination has been effective in slowing progression of kidney disease in patients with diabetes and in non-diabetic patients with proteinuria (≥200 mg/g). Both KDIGO and KDOQI recommend that the target blood pressure be less than 130/80 mm Hg for all patients with kidney disease but the JNC 8 recommends less than 140/90 mm Hg for patients younger than 60 years with kidney disease and diabetes.

36. C: The KDIGO lipid guidelines recommend treatment with a statin or statin/ezetimibe combination for all patients 50 years and younger with eGFR <60 mL/min/1.73 m² and not on dialysis. Those who are 50 years and older at stage 1 or 2 of chronic kidney disease and eGFR ≥60 mL/min/1.73 m² should be treated with a statin only but not the combination drugs. Those who are younger than 50 years and not on dialysis should be treated with a statin if they are have a risk of cardiovascular disease greater than 10% (such as those with diabetes or coronary artery disease).

37. D: Before therapy with an erythropoiesis-stimulating agent (ESA) is initiated in patients with chronic kidney disease, iron status should be assessed, along with iron bioavailability. About 40% of nondialytic patients with chronic kidney disease exhibit iron deficiency anemia, which is believed to be a precipitating factor in ESA resistance, so correcting iron status is important before beginning ESA treatment. If ESA resistance occurs (no increase in hemoglobin after 1 month of ESA treatment), then the cause of resistance must be identified.

38. A: The transferrin saturation test is transferrin saturation (%) = (serum iron level X 100)/total iron binding capacity. If the level falls below 20%, then the bioavailability is insufficient, and this may result in decreased effectiveness of ESA therapy. Serum ferritin, also commonly monitored, provides information about how much iron is stored, but the result may be affected by chronic inflammation. Low levels of albumin are also associated with hyporesponsiveness of ESA therapy, and concentration of albumin correlates with hemoglobin so that when albumin levels increase, hemoglobin tends to increase as well.

39. B: If a nondialytic patient with chronic kidney disease requires treatment for iron deficiency anemia, KDIGO recommends oral iron supplements as initial therapy. IV iron infusions may be necessary if response is not adequate after 1 to 3 months of oral supplements. If IV infusion is indicated, then low-molecular-weight iron (dextrans, ferrous gluconate, iron sucrose, or ferumoxytol) is recommended over high-molecular-weight iron, which has a higher risk of precipitating an anaphylactic reaction.

40. C: Kidney failure is generally considered inevitable when loss of kidney function reaches 50% to 60%. Patients may stabilize if treatment is able to reverse some of the kidney damage before patients lose 40% to 50% of kidney function. As nephrons are lost, hyperfiltration occurs in the remaining glomeruli in order to increase the GFR, but this causes stress and damage to the glomeruli. If this downward spiral continues, the patient will develop ESKD.

41. B: If a high-pressure alarm for arterial pressure (pre-pump) sounds during hemodialysis, this could indicate a drop in the blood pump speed. The alarm could also indicate separation of the bloodline (with upper limit set below zero), a leak between access site and monitoring site, as well as infusion of drugs or normal saline. A low-pressure alarm for arterial pressure may indicate vasoconstriction, a kink in the arterial bloodline, a poorly functioning central catheter, hypotension, infiltration of the arterial needle, or blockage of blood flow from the arterial access site.

42. B: Because sexual dysfunction is a common occurrence with chronic kidney disease and renal failure, the nurse should likely initially discuss this issue if the patient expresses concern about the effect that his disease will have on his marriage and relationship with his spouse. Patients may be embarrassed to ask about sexual dysfunction directly but can benefit from a frank discussion, including information about resources available to the patient and his spouse. If possible, the patient's spouse should be included in the discussion.

43. C: The cardiac abnormality that is most prevalent in patients with chronic kidney disease and renal failure is left ventricular hypertrophy, with the prevalence increasing in direct proportion to the stage of renal failure. Even patients in the beginning stages often exhibit LVH with 50% to 80% exhibiting LVH at the time that dialysis is initiated. Patients are at increased risk of mortality associated with cardiovascular disease, which accounts for at least half of the deaths of patients with chronic kidney disease.

Section Description: Novak Case Questions

44. C: Sodium modeling may be indicated for a patient who routinely develops hypotension during hemodialysis. Sodium modeling occurs when the sodium level in the dialysate is higher at the beginning of treatment than it is later in the treatment so that the patient's sodium level returns to normal at the end of treatment. The higher the sodium content, the more fluid that is drawn from the tissues into the blood. However, sodium modeling makes some patients thirstier so that they drink more, and this in turn can result in increased blood pressure.

45. D: If a patient on hemodialysis has a blood flow rate of 400 and the serum urea nitrogen is 100 at inflow and 35 at outflow, the urea reduction ratio (URR) expressed in percentages is 65%. The formula for URR is:
- (inflow – outflow/100) X 100.
- (100 -35/100) X 100 = 65%.

The URR is used to estimate the amount of urea nitrogen that is removed from the blood by dialysis. The goal is usually about a 65% reduction.

46. A: If the nurse has calculated the target weight loss for a patient's hemodialysis session, but the patient insists that the nurse has made an error and that the target is 1 kg too high,

the nurse should recalculate the target weight loss with the patient to determine which target is correct. Patients should be taught to monitor their own care because anyone can make mistakes, and patients often are very knowledgeable about their conditions and needs.

47. B: Weight gain between hemodialysis treatments should not exceed 5% of dry weight. One kilogram (2.2 lb) of increased weight represents 1 liter of fluid retention. Dry weight is the optimal post-dialysis weight after excess fluid has been removed. Because patients may gain weight because of the glucose in dialysate solutions or lose weight because of lost muscle mass or fat stores, it is important to reevaluate the patient's dry weight at least every 2 weeks to ensure adequate removal of excess fluids.

48. C: The target for serum ferritin for patients on hemodialysis is ≥200 ng/mL. Adults with normal kidney function usually are not diagnosed with iron deficiency anemia if their serum ferritin level is greater than 15 ng/mL. However, the targets are higher with patients with chronic kidney disease because the inflammation associated with kidney disease increases the level of serum ferritin, so ≥100 ng/mL is recommended as the target for patients with chronic kidney disease and ≥200 ng/mL for patients on hemodialysis.

49. B: When calculating the amount of fluid that must be removed during dialysis, fluid to offset the patient's weight gain must be included (1 kg = 1000 mL). Added to this is the volume of saline used to prime the system, any medications added in liquid form, the saline used to clear the system at the completion of the treatment and any fluids ingested during treatment. This would include fluids, such as coffee or water, and ice chips.

50. C: If a patient with adult-onset polycystic kidney disease asks the nurse what the chance is that the disease will pass to any children if the patient's spouse is disease free, the nurse should advise the patient that a child will have a 50% risk of developing the disease. Polycystic kidney disease is an autosomal dominant disorder that usually remains latent until the third or fourth decade of life and involves both kidneys with the cortex and medulla filling with multiple large cysts that destroy the kidney tissue.

Section Description: Rodriguez Case Questions

51. D: Calcium channel blockers may result in cloudy peritoneal fluid for patients on peritoneal dialysis, possibly because the calcium channel blockers result in increased concentration of triglycerides in the solution. While cloudy peritoneal solution is often indicative of infection (cell counts >50 to 100/mcL), it can also indicate increased levels of monocytes or eosinophils without peritonitis. Peritoneal solution may also become cloudy in the presence of malignancy, blood, or fibrin, and may appear cloudy after an extended dwell period.

52. A: Spiking of dialysis bags places the patient with peritoneal dialysis at high risk for peritonitis because the system can easily be contaminated if aseptic technique is broken. For this reason, closed systems are preferable. The "flush before fill" procedure helps to reduce risk of contamination. Other risk factors include single-cuff catheters and upward directed exit sites (these should be directed downward or laterally). Hypokalemia also places patients at increased risk of enteric peritonitis.

53. B: If a patient's peritoneal catheter cultures positive for fungal organisms, indicating that the catheter is colonized, the most likely intervention is removal of the catheter and

temporary hemodialysis, allowing the peritoneum to rest, along with antifungals as indicated. Once a catheter is colonized, there is little chance that it can be saved. The patient may require hemodialysis for a number of months to ensure that the fungal infection is eradicated before another peritoneal catheter is inserted.

54. C: When patients are undergoing peritoneal dialysis, the most common pathway of infection resulting in peritonitis is intraluminal, usually from poor technique that allows bacteria to enter the system. The most common organisms are coagulase-negative staphylococci or diphtheroids. Other pathways include periluminal from bacteria present on the skin, hematogenous from distant infections, transvaginal from organisms migrating up the uterus and fallopian tubes to the peritoneum, and transmural from organisms migrating from the bowel wall (often associated with colonoscopy or diarrhea states).

55. B: If a patient on CAPD requires a sample of peritoneal solution for evaluation of the cell count, the correct method of obtaining the specimen is to invert the drainage bag a few times to make sure the solution is well mixed and then to aspirate a sample from the bag port. A sample is obtained directly from the peritoneal catheter only in patients who are "day dry" but may have some fluid remaining in the abdomen. Careful aseptic technique must be followed to prevent contamination.

56. C: If a sample of peritoneal fluid cannot be immediately processed, the inoculated culture bottles should ideally be stored at 37 °C. The sample should be immediately placed into the EDTA-containing tube because delay of 3 to 5 hours may result in the inability to identify cell types. Prolonged storage may result in growth of pathogenic organisms. A minimum of 50 mL of fluid should be obtained for the specimen to increase the likelihood of a positive culture.

Section Description: Independent Questions, Group 2

57. B: The most important factor in preventing exsanguination from dialysis line separation is access site visibility. Because the blood is pumped through the system at the rate of 350 mL/min up to 500 mL/min, the patient can lose total volume of blood within 10 minutes. While patient education is important, patients often fall asleep during treatment. Venous needle dislodgment is not always detected by alarms, so one should not rely on alarms solely. HemaClips are important safety additions, but should not replace observation.

58. B: The 3 bloodborne pathogens that pose the most risk for hemodialysis patients are hepatitis B, hepatitis C, and HIV. Hepatitis B is highly contagious and may be spread from contaminated vials, surfaces, and drugs, as well as from individuals who are infected. Patients should be advised to have the hepatitis B vaccination to protect them from infection. Hepatitis C spreads less readily than hepatitis B but still poses risk. HIV is also spread through blood and body fluids.

59. A: If a patient has pain and tightness in the chest with pain radiation to the jaw and down the left arm, the nurse's immediate intervention should be to slow the blood flow rate to 150 mL/min because this decreases the amount of stress on the heart. The ultrafiltration rate should also be decreased to slow loss of fluid as this may further stress the heart. The patient's vital signs should be assessed and the physician notified. If the patient is hypotensive, then a bolus of saline is indicated. Oxygen may be administered if the patient is dyspneic.

60. C: The potassium level in dialysate is commonly 2 mM. If the patient's potassium level is less than 4.5 mEq/L, then the potassium level of the dialysate may be increased to 3 mM, although patients may require sodium polystyrene sulfonate resin (Kayexalate) to prevent hyperkalemia during treatment. Dialysate with 1 mM potassium should be used only for very short periods because this level has been associated with increased risk of cardiac arrest.

61. A: The first step in the Continuous Quality Improvement (CQI) process is to identify the need for improvement, and this could be a major or minor problem. Once this is identified, then the process must be analyzed through the work of a team that reviews data, studies the problems, and identifies patterns or trends. This usually entails conducting a root cause analysis to determine where the process has failed. The last step is to carry out the plan-do-check-act (PDCA) cycle.

62. A: The 2 hormones secreted by the kidneys are erythropoietin and calcitriol. Erythropoietin stimulates the bone marrow to increase production of red blood cells. Without adequate erythropoietin, the patient develops anemia; therefore, erythropoiesis-stimulating agent (ESA) may be ordered to increase red blood cell production. Calcitriol is derived from calciferol, which is synthesized by the skin after exposure to ultraviolet light or ingested in the diet (as from vitamin D–enriched dairy products). The liver converts calciferol to vitamin D3, which is converted to calcitriol by the kidneys. Calcitriol promotes absorption of calcium and phosphate.

63. B: When instructing a patient on hemodialysis about weight gain, the patient should be advised that the usual goal for interdialytic weight gain is less than 1 kg per day; it is common for patients to gain more than this amount. If weight gain is excessive, patients should be cautioned about limiting sodium intake, as this restriction is usually more important than fluid restriction as increased sodium increases thirst.

64. A: If a patient has itching and stuffy nose that usually occurs only during hemodialysis, the most likely cause is hypersensitivity reaction, usually to dialyzer or blood circuit components. Reactions to dialyzers are most common with new dialyzers ("first-use syndrome") and may range from mild allergic response to anaphylaxis. Although reusable dialyzers are carefully processed and rinsed before reuse, some sterilants, which may cause allergic responses, may remain.

65. B: If an elderly patient undergoing hemodialysis has expressed the wish to die but never requested a DNR order and experiences a cardiac arrest, the correct initial response is to carry out CPR and defibrillation. Patients often express the wish to die, and they have the right to refuse treatment and request no life-saving treatments. However, since the patient did not request a DNR order, nursing staff cannot assume that the patient would want no resuscitation efforts made.

66. D: During hemodialysis, if a patient who is lying in supine position has chest pain, begins coughing, and shows evidence of cyanosis of distal extremities and lips, the nurse should suspect that the patient has air embolism. In supine recumbent position, the air often enters the heart (as opposed to the brain if the patient is sitting upright), generating foam in the right ventricle and into the lungs. If air returns from the lungs to the left atrium and

ventricle, it can enter the arterial system and cause severe cardiac and neurological impairment.

67. A: Marked eosinophilia in a patient undergoing hemodialysis puts the patient at increased risk of type A (anaphylactic) dialyzer reaction. The reason for eosinophilia in patients with kidney disease is not clear, but there is some indication that eosinophilia is more associated with vascular disease, such as may occur with diabetes, than uremia. Studies have shown that eosinophil counts drop during the first quarter hour of dialysis and then increase markedly at the end of the dialysis session.

68. D: If severe hemolysis occurs during hemodialysis, the patient is at risk for hyperkalemia because potassium is released when red blood cells are hemolyzed. Hyperkalemia can lead to cardiac abnormalities and cardiac arrest, so the blood pump should be stopped immediately so that blood with high levels of potassium is not reinfused into the patient. The patient may need treatment for both hyperkalemia as well as a drop in hematocrit because of the volume of blood that cannot be reinfused.

69. B: The purpose of a "zero lift" program is to prevent injuries, most commonly musculoskeletal disorders involving damage to muscles, nerves, and tendons. While staff can still assist patients to move and ambulate, staff members should avoid manual lifting as much as possible. It is important when instituting a "zero lift" program that staff members are trained in alternate methods, such as the use of assistive devices, and that the necessary equipment is readily available.

70. C: The legal document that assigns a healthcare proxy to make decisions in the event that a person is unable to do so is a durable power of attorney. Legal requirements vary from one state to another, and in some cases, an advance directive may contain a durable power of attorney or may designate an individual to make decisions about health care. A living will is similar to an advance directive and outlines the type of care the patient desires if the patient is dying or unconscious. A DNR (do-not-resuscitate) order specifies the condition under which the patient does not want to be resuscitated.

71. D: If the administration of a dialysis center bills for good and services that were not provided, it can be prosecuted under the False Claims Act, which prohibits any false claims to the United States if the person submitting the claim understands that it is fraudulent. Other actions that are prohibited include billing for goods or services that were unnecessary, billing for services that were provided but were substandard, accepting or giving kickbacks, and unbundling of charges for supplies or services that should be grouped.

72. D: Because of the interdisciplinary care needed by most hemodialysis patients, the first step when utilizing the "Got Chart" method of contacting a physician by telephone is to ensure the nurse is contacting the correct physician (nephrologist, primary care physician, consultant). Before completing the call, the nurse should check recent progress notes, standing orders, and physician preferences regarding how, when, and where to call. Additionally, the nurse should determine if the physician needs to be consulted about any other patient to avoid extra calls. The telephoning nurse should personally assess the patient before calling.

73. D: When utilizing Maslow's Hierarchy of Needs to set priorities in nursing care for hemodialysis patients, that level of needs that has the highest priority is physiologic, which

includes the need for oxygen, food, elimination, control of temperature, sex, movement, rest, and comfort. The next level of concern is that of safety and security, followed by love and belonging, and self-esteem. Self-actualization is the highest level and is often dependent on meeting needs at the lower levels.

Section Description: Mason Case Questions

74. D: The purpose of "vessel mapping" is to ensure that the physician will find adequate vessels for the AV fistula. Vessel mapping utilizes Doppler ultrasound to assess vessels. The normal rate of blood flow in the brachial artery in a patient with end-stage kidney disease is less than 100 mL/min, but the AV fistula must be able to accommodate much higher volumes (up to 1200 mL/min for radiocephalic fistula and up to 1500 mL/min for brachiocephalic fistula), so choosing a vessel that can dilate sufficiently is critical.

75. C: When determining if a new AV fistula is maturing, the 3 factors assessed by palpation are the thrill, vessel growth, and vessel firmness. The thrill should not have the character of a pulse but should be a constant vibratory sensation. The vessel should begin to grow soon after surgery and should be evident by 2 weeks. The growth should be assessed for evenness and any flat spots, which may indicate stenosis, should be noted. The vessel should become firmer as the vessel becomes stronger.

76. C: Nighttime hemodialysis with 7- to 8-hour sessions 3 times weekly has a number of advantages, including a better survival rate, because patients have about twice as many hours of dialysis compared with the usual daytime schedule (3 times a week for 3 to 4 hours). Patients also have fewer food and fluid restrictions. Patients have fewer complications because the slower hemodialysis is less damaging to the cardiovascular system and removes more of the β-2 M protein that causes amyloidosis.

77. A: Patients should be advised to avoid eating during hemodialysis because ingestion of food may result in hypotension. Patients who tend to be hypotensive during hemodialysis should also avoid eating immediately before the treatment. Eating likely causes dilation of the splanchnic venous system and reduces circulating volume of blood. This effect may continue for up to 2 hours after eating. Oral fluids should also be limited or avoided because it can take up to 10 hours for the fluids to be absorbed into the systemic circulation.

78. C: The most important reason for placing hemodialysis needles in antegrade position is because it causes less scarring than the retrograde position. When a needle is placed in antegrade position, the blood flows in the direction of the needle so that the blood flow will hold the small flap created by the needle closed. If the needle is in retrograde position, the needle points in the opposite direction of the blood flow, so when the needle is removed, the blood flow keeps the flap open.

79. D: If a patient receiving hemodialysis has weakness, and the nurse notes increasing muscle atrophy of the legs, decreased range of motion, and difficulty walking, the nurse should ask the physician to refer the patient for physical therapy. While general fatigues and weakness may prevent some patients from participating in physical therapy, this patient may benefit from strengthening exercises and a walking or cycling program. The physical therapist can evaluate the patient's physical abilities and determine an appropriate program.

80. B: If a patient on hemodialysis persists in smoking despite attempts to educate him about the risks of smoking, the nurse should advise the patient that nicotine levels after smoking are higher in dialysis patients than in people without kidney disease. Thus, the patient may experience more adverse effects than his parents or siblings, who also smoke but do not have kidney disease. Smoking increases the risk of cardiovascular disease, which is the primary cause of death among patients undergoing dialysis.

81. A: If a hemodialysis patient wants to try herbal or complementary medicine to control chronic itching, the therapy that may be most beneficial is acupuncture, the use of which is supported by studies showing that acupuncture provided some relief of symptoms. Both acupuncture and electroacupuncture may provide some relief in the intensity of itching but may not eliminate itching. St. John's wort may react with a variety of different drugs and its safety for patients on dialysis is not clear.

82. D: If 5 minutes after initiation of a hemodialysis treatment the patient experiences dyspnea, generalized edema, tingling about the mouth, and feeling faint, and has periorbital edema and hives, the nurse should immediately call for help and clamp all lines and stop the hemodialysis. Because these symptoms are consistent with anaphylaxis, blood in the system should not be returned to the patient as this may increase the allergic response. Oxygen may be administered to relieve dyspnea. Epinephrine may be administered to control anaphylaxis.

Section Description: Walker Case Questions

83. C: Ideally, for a patient with chronic kidney disease and one who will eventually have to have hemodialysis, a phlebotomist should draw blood from the hand veins to avoid trauma to the veins in the arms, which must be preserved for access sites. PICC lines should also be avoided as they may cause scarring that results in outflow problems. Drawing blood from foot veins should be done only if no other access is available because of increased risk of complications.

84. D: A patient with chronic kidney disease should have an AV fistula created 6 to 9 months prior to the expected onset of dialysis because of the prolonged period needed for healing of the AV fistula. Additionally, finding adequate veins may be difficult in patients with chronic inflammation and cardiovascular disease, commonly found with patients with kidney disease. Additionally, an AV fistula may not function properly, so a second AV fistula may need to be created.

85. C: Dialysis is usually started in a patient with chronic kidney disease when the patient's eGFR falls to about 8 mL/min/1.73 m^2. Patients usually begin to exhibit signs of uremia when the level falls to about 7 L/min/1.73 m^2. The patient should be carefully assessed and monitored when levels fall to 10 to 12 mL/min/1.73 m^2 because some patients, depending on symptoms (such as fluid retention), may require onset of dialysis before the rate falls to 8 mL/min/1.73 m^2.

86. C: If the patient's PTH level is high, the most appropriate referral is likely to an endocrinologist. It can be challenging to manage PTH levels and to accurately titrate medications, such as cinacalcet and vitamin D, in order to prevent further complications. If the patient has diabetes, she may already be under the care of an endocrinologist to manage

the diabetes. Disease management for the patient with chronic kidney disease often requires multidisciplinary effort.

87. B: Patients with severe kidney disease should avoid MRI with gadolinium contrast agent because it may result in nephrogenic systemic fibrosis, which causes fibrosis of the skin as well as internal organs (similar to scleroderma) and for which there is no treatment. If a patient with kidney disease absolutely must have gadolinium contrast agent because of inability to tolerate other imaging procedures, then the lowest possible dose of gadolinium contrast should be used, and the patient may need to undergo temporary hemodialysis after the MRI to ensure rapid removal of the contrast agent.

88. C: When teaching a patient with chronic kidney disease about dietary restrictions, the patient should be advised to limit dietary phosphorus intake to 800 to 1000 mg/day in order to maintain a normal phosphorus level of 2.5 to 4.5 mg/dL. Foods and fluids high in phosphorus include chocolate, dark colas, dairy products, organ meats, sardines, oysters, dried beans and peas, nuts, whole grains, bran, and seeds. Patients may be prescribed phosphate binders to absorb some of the phosphorus from foods.

89. D: According to KDOQI guidelines, patients with chronic kidney disease should restrict calcium intake to 2000 mg/day. Some authorities recommend a lower limit of 1500 mg/day in order to keep the serum calcium level in the low to mid-normal range as a means of reducing the risk of vascular calcification. If the patient is taking calcium-based phosphorus binders, this calcium must be added to the dietary intake of calcium. Many foods high in calcium (such as dairy products) are also high in phosphorus and should be avoided.

90. B: In a patient with chronic kidney disease, metabolic acidosis results in increased reabsorption of bone and may also increase the progression of kidney disease. The serum bicarbonate level should be maintained at 22 mmol/L or higher. Treatment to prevent metabolic acidosis is sodium bicarbonate at 0.5 to 1 mmol/kg per day in order to prevent reabsorption of bone. Metabolic acidosis becomes acute when the GFR decreases to about 20 mL/min because the kidneys can no longer filter acids adequately.

91. A: If a patient is taking cyclosporine as an antirejection drug after kidney transplant, but states that his general practitioner is concerned about his cholesterol level and has ordered atorvastatin, the nurse should call the physician to discuss possible adverse interactions. When a patient takes both cyclosporine and atorvastatin, the combination can increase the blood levels of the statin drug, increasing the risk of myopathy and rhabdomyolysis. Generally, this combination should be avoided, but if so ordered, the patient must be very carefully monitored, and the dosage of the atorvastatin may need to be decreased.

92. A: Following kidney transplantation and initiation of immunosuppression, the viral infection that is usually the most cause for concern is cytomegalovirus (CMV). Viral infections usually occur after the first month with 20% to 60% of kidney recipients developing CMV infection. CMV has immunomodulating effects and can result in vascular damage, both of which may increase the risk of graft failure. Patients are often treated prophylactically with an antiviral medication, such as ganciclovir, to prevent CMV infection.

93. A: MRSA infection is a healthcare-associated infection that usually occurs within the first month of surgery because of contact with the bacteria in the immediate postoperative period. Other infections that may occur include vancomycin-resistant enterococci (VRE),

Candida spp., and *Clostridium difficile*. Patients may also develop infections from the donor organ but this is uncommon. These infections include HSV, HIV, West Nile, *Trypanosoma cruzi,* and rabies. Patients may also develop infection from their own colonized bacteria, including *Aspergillus* and *Pseudomonas.*

94. C: If a patient who received a kidney transplantation adheres closely to treatment regimens for the first 10 months and then begins missing physician appointments and failing to take all of prescribed medications, stating that he is doing fine and does not need to follow such a strict regimen, the defense mechanism the patient is using is denial. Denial is very common once patients have to live with the reality of an organ transplant and the immunosuppression required.

Section Description: Independent Questions, Group 3

95. D: When considering the chain of infection, the 3 most common reservoirs of interest include humans, environment, and animals. Humans are the most common reservoir associated with healthcare-associated infections. The human reservoir may have an acute or subacute infection or may be a carrier with no personal sign of infection. A nasal carrier, for example, may spread *Staphylococcus aureus* to other patients without any sign of infection. In the prodromal stage of some infections, the human reservoir may show no signs of infection. With some infection, the human reservoir may have recovered but is still shedding bacteria.

96. D: Immunoglobulins are proteins or antibodies that provide a defense against various antigens. Immunoglobulin G (IgG) is the primary circulating interstitial antibody, found in all body fluids, including plasma, and helps protect the body against both viral and bacterial infections. IgG, which easily enters tissue, is the primary immunoglobulin to protect tissue and the most abundant immunoglobulin. IgG occurs late in an immune response but survives longer than other immunoglobulins. There are 4 subtypes of IgG: IgG1, IgG2, IgG3, and IgG4.

97. C: The primary reason that some hospital units ban fresh flowers and plants is that they may carry pathogenic organisms, including antibiotic-resistant organisms that are implicated in outbreaks. Most bans cover units with critically ill patients, such as intensive care units or transplant units, but some hospitals ban flowers and plants in all areas of the hospital. If flowers are allowed, then the water should be changed by housekeeping staff and not nursing staff with patient contact because hands may become contaminated when changing water.

98. A: If 4 patients on a hospital unit develop infections with *Clostridium difficile* in 1 week, this would be classified as an outbreak. Epidemic has essentially the same meaning—an increase in infections over the number predicted—but the term epidemic is usually used to denote a more widespread outbreak, usually with many cases in a wider area. Outbreaks are common in hospitals and often are associated with breaks in protocol, such as with inadequate handwashing.

99. A: When an increase in infections occurs in a hospital unit, besides notifying the administration (which can in turn notify risk management and public affairs), the hospital unit that should also be notified is the microbiology laboratory so that it can be on alert for further indications of infection. The laboratory should save any isolates that may be part of

the outbreak to help with tracing the origins of the outbreak. The laboratory should be in direct communication with infection prevention professionals.

100. D: If there is an outbreak of *Aspergillus* infections in a hemodialysis center, an outbreak investigation should include review of construction projects in or near patient areas. *Aspergillus* spores are typically inhaled. *Aspergillus* infections are often associated with construction projects, which release the spores. These projects may even be outside of the facility, such as in an adjacent property, especially if windows are open or air filters become contaminated. Air-conditioning systems may also become contaminated, especially those placed in windows.

101. C: The number one cause of kidney failure in the United States is diabetes mellitus, type 2, accounting for about 40% of the overall cases. Type 1 diabetes (which is less common) results in about 4% of the total. Because some ethnic groups, such as African Americans, Native Americans, and Hispanics, have high rates of diabetes, they are also at increased risk of kidney failure. Diabetes causes cardiovascular changes, and the changes in the small vessels in the kidney impair its ability to function.

102. C: If the patient cannot tolerate contrast for a CT and needs an MRI to evaluate a mass on his kidney, cancelling the MRI is not a viable solution. When patients are very claustrophobic, reassuring them or advising them to practice relaxation is not likely to be effective, so the best solution is likely to contact the physician and request an order for a sedative. Generally, when patients require sedation to relieve anxiety, alprazolam (Xanax) is the medication of choice and is usually administered immediately before the procedure.

103. A: A specific gravity of less than 1.01 may produce a false-negative finding in a urine dipstick for protein because the urine is dilute. Other factors that may result in a false negative are urine that has a high sodium content, urine that is acidic, and the presence of nonalbumin proteinuria because the dipsticks detect albumin. Other factors may also result in a false positive. These include the presence of blood or semen in the sample, urine that is alkaline, contamination of the sample with detergents, disinfectants, or radiocontrast agents, as well as a specific gravity of greater than 1.03.

104. C: Anaphylaxis may result in ischemic injury to the kidneys. With ischemia, the inadequate perfusion results in impaired tubular endothelial function and damage to tubular cells as well as cast formation. Other causes of ischemic injury include hemorrhage, volume depletion, prolonged hypotension, shock (cardiogenic, hypovolemic, and septic), and sepsis. Nephrotoxic causes of kidney injury include endogenous toxins from rhabdomyolysis and tumor lysis syndrome, antimicrobials, immunosuppressants, chemotherapeutics, illicit drugs (heroin, PCP, and amphetamines), and NSAIDs.

105. D: According to the Renal Physicians Association's clinical practice guidelines to determine if dialysis should be avoided or stopped in patients with end-stage kidney disease, one requirement is shared decision making. Patients (and family) should be fully informed about the disease and should have advance planning. Forgoing dialysis may be considered for patients with poor prognosis or with marked risk factors. A process should be in place for conflict resolution in case of disagreement, and palliative services should be available.

106. B: Prostatic hypertrophy is an example of a post-renal cause of acute kidney injury, which is an obstruction in the urinary tract below the kidney, such as in the ureter or the bladder neck, making the urine back up into the kidney. Prerenal causes of acute kidney injury are those conditions that decrease perfusion of the kidney before the arterial blood reaches the kidney. Intrarenal causes are those that produce injury through ischemia or toxins inside the kidney at the nephrons.

107. A: Sepsis that is associated with renal ischemia may result in acute tubular necrosis, the most common cause of acute kidney injury. The 3 primary causes of acute tubular necrosis are ischemia, sepsis, and nephrotoxins. Ischemia results in damage to the basement membrane and damage to the tubular epithelium while nephrotoxins result in necrosis of the tubular epithelial cells, which in turn obstructs the tubules. This condition may be reversible if treated promptly.

108. A: Although the patient's laboratory results show multiple abnormalities, the priority for intervention is the elevated potassium because hyperkalemia puts the patient at risk for cardiac dysrhythmias and cardiac arrest, and the patient is nearing the critical value. Potassium values:
- Normal values: 3.5 to 5.5 mEq/L.
- Hypokalemia: <3.5 mEq/L. Critical value: <2.5 mEq/L.
- Hyperkalemia: >5.5 mEq/L. Critical value: >6.5 mEq/L.

109. D: Calcium carbonate can bind to iron polysaccharide complex and decrease the effectiveness of the iron, so they should not be given together. At least 2 hours should separate administration of the medications. Oral iron polysaccharide complex is given to patients with kidney failure to increase iron level because epoetin alfa cannot produce hemoglobin without adequate iron stores. Calcium is used to bind with phosphorus to decrease serum phosphorus levels and to compensate for a diet low in dairy products.

110. B: Aluminum hydroxide may increase the risk of osteomalacia and refractory anemia in a patient with chronic kidney disease and may also result in encephalopathy if aluminum toxicity occurs. Aluminum hydroxide is a phosphorus binder that prevents intestinal absorption of phosphorus, thereby decreasing serum phosphorus and increasing serum calcium. Because of the problems associated with toxicity, aluminum hydroxide is usually avoided and replaced with calcium binders. Aluminum hydroxide may interact with numerous other medications.

111. C: If a patient with chronic kidney disease on dialysis has been prescribed cinacalcet (Sensipar), this probably indicates that the patient has elevated parathyroid hormone, as secondary hyperparathyroidism is common with chronic kidney disease. Cinacalcet is usually indicated when PTH levels increase to 3 times normal range. Treatment, however, puts the patient at risk of hypocalcemia and adynamic bone disease (especially if PTH falls below 100 pg/mL). Calcium and phosphorus levels should be carefully monitored during treatment with cinacalcet.

112. D: If, when percussing the right kidney area of a patient using indirect fist percussion, the patient experiences pain when the nurse delivers a firm blow, this likely indicates kidney infection or polycystic kidney disease, as this procedure should not elicit pain. Because patient did experience pain, further tests, such as laboratory tests and imaging, are indicated to determine the cause. The nurse should also palpate the kidneys to determine if

they are enlarged, although the left kidney is usually not palpable because of the position of the spleen.

113. D: If a 24-hour urine quantitative protein test shows persistent proteinuria, this usually indicates glomerular renal disease. Protein found in the urine is usually albumin. A 24-hour test should result in fewer than 150 mg of protein. Glomerular renal disease interferes with the kidneys' ability to filter toxins so that some toxins that should be excreted are retained in the blood, and proteins and red blood cells that should be retained are excreted in the urine.

114. B: Following a renal biopsy, a compression bandage should be applied to the needle insertion site and the patient should be positioned on biopsy side for up to 60 minutes and bedrest for 24 hours. The biopsy is usually done in the lower lobe of the kidney percutaneously and may be done with CT or ultrasound guidance. Following the biopsy, the patient should be assessed for hypotension, flank pain, increasing temperature, chills, dysuria, and bleeding.

115. B: With the autosomal recessive form of medullary cystic disease, kidney failure usually occurs before 20 years of age. With the autosomal dominant disease, kidney failure usually occurs after age 30. Cysts form in the medulla of the kidney, resulting in asymmetric kidneys that are grossly scarred, interfering with the ability of the kidneys to concentrate urine. Symptoms include polyuria, metabolic acidosis, hyponatremia, hypertension, anemia, and progressive kidney failure.

Section Description: Santos Case Questions

116. C: If, following treatment for leukemia, a patient develops tumor lysis syndrome, cell lysis results in hyperuricemia, which in turn causes urinary obstruction because the increased levels of uric acid result in metabolic acidosis and crystallization of the uric acid in the kidneys. The kidneys are unable to adequately filter the crystals and the GFR decreases, resulting in renal insufficiency and acute kidney failure. Calcium and phosphorus ions bind and create calcium phosphate salts, which then precipitate in the renal tubules, increasing the risk of inflammation and obstruction.

117. A: The electrolyte imbalances that are likely to occur with tumor lysis syndrome are:
- Hyperkalemia: Intracellular K is rapidly expelled into the systemic circulation, resulting in muscular and cardiac abnormalities.
- Hyperphosphatemia: Intracellular PO_4 is released, resulting in muscle cramping tetany, cardiac dysrhythmias, and seizures.
- Hypocalcemia: Calcium levels fall as calcium and phosphorus bind, forming calcium phosphate, resulting in muscle cramping, tetany, cardiac dysrhythmias, and renal failure from acute nephrocalcinosis.

118. C: If a patient requires treatment for hyperuricemia to prevent uric acid crystallization, an alkalinizing agent is administered. Commonly used medications include allopurinol, acetazolamide (Diamox), and sodium bicarbonate. Acetazolamide increases urinary pH by decreasing resorption of bicarbonate in the proximal tubules. Sodium bicarbonate alkalinizes the urine (target is 7) to increase the solubility of uric acid. Use of sodium bicarbonate must include careful monitoring of urinary pH.

Section Description: Chan Case Questions

119. C: When discussing disease progression with a patient with chronic kidney disease, kidney transplantation should be initially considered at stage 4 of chronic kidney disease as this is the time when the patient should be preparing for dialysis or transplantation and making decisions about the best option. Preemptive transplantation (done without beginning dialysis) offers superior outcomes to transplantation done later, although not all patients are candidates for transplantation and kidneys may not always be readily available.

120. C: The Mini-Mental State Examination is often used as a baseline evaluation of mental status for patients who are candidates for transplant as well as donor candidates. A score of 24 or higher is within normal limits. The Mini-Mental State Examination assesses orientation (time, date, place), registration (repeating names of common objects), attention (spelling "world" backward) and calculation, recall (report common objects named earlier), and language (repeating words, following directions), with maximum scores for each task ranging from 1 to 5.

121. A: When considering whether a potential unrelated kidney donor is acceptable, the fact that the potential donor has made repeated reports about donating on multiple social media sites should be cause for concern because people who want to donate to gain publicity may have unrealistic expectations of the recipient and others. While one early episode of depression may not eliminate a person from consideration, serious or ongoing psychiatric problems may. Donors should have the cognitive ability to completely understand what is entailed in donation, and there should be no suggestion of coercion.

122. A: Following a kidney transplant, if a patient becomes agitated and confused with periods of lucidity, typical of delirium, the initial response should be reorientation and comfort measures, such as reducing light and sound and providing a sitter to stay with the patient if a family member is not available. While haloperidol may be used to reduce severe symptoms, there is some concern about using medication because studies indicate increased mortality rates for patients treated with antipsychotics.

123. D: If a patient on renal transplant medications has been experiencing visual hallucinations, the medication that is most likely the cause is cyclosporine, which may cause numerous adverse neuropsychiatric effects, including anxiety, delirium, tremors, seizures, paresthesia, and cortical blindness. More common adverse reactions include tarry or clay-colored stools; anorexia; abdominal, back, or chest pain; fever; headache; itching; nausea and vomiting; rash; ataxia; and jaundice. Patients should be advised of potential adverse effects and advised to notify healthcare providers immediately if any occur.

124. B: Patients taking cyclosporine for renal transplant medication are usually advised to avoid grapefruit and foods high in potassium, such as bananas and raisins. Patients who are also taking ACE inhibitors are especially at risk for hyperkalemia, so potassium levels should be carefully monitored. Cyclosporine may interact with numerous other drugs, so any new prescriptions should be checked against the list. Oral solutions should not be administered in plastic containers because the medication binds to plastic.

125. D: For the immediate postoperative period following kidney transplantation, patients should be advised to have a fairly high daily protein in order to promote healing, usually 1.3 to 1.5 g/kg per day. Some patients, such as those who develop infection or fever, may be

advised to increase protein intake further, up to 2 g/kg. With increased protein, patients should have intake of 30 to 35 calories/kg to avoid a negative nitrogen balance.

Section Description: Stein Case Questions

126. A: When assessing an 80-year-old patient for kidney function, the nurse expects age-related changes to result in decreased kidney size, decreased creatinine clearance, and increased BUN and serum creatinine. The kidney becomes smaller in size and weight and up to half of the glomeruli no longer function. Because of fewer functioning nephrons and decreased function in the loop of Henle and tubes, the creatinine clearance decreases and the BUN and serum creatinine increase. Urine is less concentrated because kidneys concentrate urine less efficiently.

127. B: Stage 3 chronic kidney disease is characterized by an eGFR of 30 to 59 mL/min. Stage 3 is common in older adults with other disorders, such as cardiovascular disease, and at increased risk of cardiovascular events, such as myocardial infarction or stroke. At this stage, creatinine is usually within normal limits. Many patients will stabilize at stage 3 but some will progress to ESKD. Indications that kidney disease is progressing include decreasing eGFR, proteinuria, and hematuria.

128. A: For elderly patients with chronic kidney disease who do not exhibit marked fluid overload, the need for dialysis may be delayed up to 1 year with protein restriction (very low protein diet with 0.3 to 0.6 g/kg/d) and ketoacids as well as essential amino acids to compensate for the low protein diet. Studies have shown that patients have no long-term adverse effects of this regimen. Patients must be monitored carefully to ensure adherence to the dietary restrictions.

Section Description: Woods Case Questions

129. B: If a patient is a candidate for kidney transplantation, the patient must register with the Organ Procurement and Transplantation Network (OPTN), which is administered by the United Network for Organ Sharing (UNOS). The OPTN links all regional organ procurement organizations (OPOs) and transplant centers by a computer network. Patients may register with more than 1 center but may have to undergo medical evaluations at each center and will have to meet the centers' criteria.

130. D: When a patient is on the waiting list for kidney transplantation, the 3 factors evaluated to determine if a match is appropriate are the blood type, HLA factors, and antibodies. The blood types must be compatible, although immunosuppression has allowed some success with ABO incompatibility. HLA factors must be evaluated because the more they match, the better the success rate. If blood type and HLA factors are suitable, then the donor's and recipient's blood samples are mixed to determine if the recipient produces antibodies against the donor.

131. B: If a patient on the waiting list for a kidney expresses concern that the patient's insurance and available resources will not cover all of the cost of kidney transplantation, the Internet resource that may provide the most valuable information is UNOS Transplant Living. This site provides detailed information about the entire process and has a section about financing a transplant with links to various funding sources and guides for dealing with insurance and maintaining necessary records.

132. A: Age 55 at death (older than 50 years) would classify a cadaveric kidney donor as a marginal or expanded criteria donor (ECD) according to UNOS criteria. Other criteria include terminal creatinine of greater than 1.5 mg/dL, a history of diabetes mellitus, a long history of hypertension. A donor is considered marginal if stroke is the cause of death. Another important consideration is the cold ischemia time (CIT). The longer the CIT, the bigger the risk of graft failure and mortality. Although no ideal CIT has been documented, extended CITs (longer than 36 hours) are of special concern.

133. B: The primary purpose of dual kidney transplantation is to increase the success rates of marginal kidneys, especially those from older donors. Studies indicate that success rates of double kidney transplantation are equal to or superior to rates for single kidney transplantation with marginal kidneys, especially after the first year. Double kidney transplantation is one way to expand opportunities for transplantation with marginal kidneys that might otherwise be discarded because of increased risk of failure.

134. D: HLA-DR along with HLA-A and HLA-B are the 3 critical major histocompatibility complex (MHC) genes for matching donor and recipient because these genes have the greatest effect on rejection of a donor organ. Other important but less critical genes are HLA-C, HLA-DQ, and HLA-DP. The human leukocyte antigen (HLA) genes are classified as class I (HLA-A, HLA-B, and HLA-C) and class II (HLA-DP, HLA-DQ, and HLA-DR). The greater the degree of matching between donor and recipient, the less likely the patient is to experience rejection of the donor organ.

135. C: Following kidney transplantation, kidney patients are at risk for numerous types of cancer with up to 20% of patients developing cancer after 10 years. The most common cancer is skin cancer, usually non-melanoma, with squamous cell carcinoma the most frequent. The next most common cancer is renal cell carcinoma, usually developing in native kidneys rather than transplanted kidneys. Renal cell carcinoma often occurs bilaterally and may be treated with nephrectomy, total or partial.

Section Description: Independent Questions, Group 4

136. D: According to the RIFLE (**R**isk, **I**njury, **F**ailure, **L**oss, **E**nd-stage kidney disease) criteria, the Failure stage occurs with urine output less than 0.3 mL/kg/h for 24 hours (oliguria) or anuria for 12 hours. Other indications include serum creatinine increased 3 times over normal or GFR decreased by 75% or serum creatinine greater than 4 mg/dL with acute increase of at least 0.5 mg/dL. Loss is characterized by complete loss of kidney function for more than 4 weeks and end-stage kidney disease is defined as complete loss of kidney function for more than 3 months.

137. A: During the diuretic phase of acute kidney injury, the patient should be closely monitored for dehydration, hyponatremia, and hypokalemia. During this phase, the urinary output usually increases from about 1 L to 3 to 5 L per day because of osmotic diuresis. During the diuretic phase, the kidneys are able to excrete wastes but unable to concentrate urine, resulting in hypovolemia and hypotension. This phase may last for 1 to 3 weeks before the patient enters the recovery phase.

138. D: If a patient with acute kidney injury is prescribed sodium polystyrene sulfonate (Kayexalate), paralytic ileus is a contraindication because administration of the drug may

result in necrosis of intestinal tissue. Sodium polystyrene sulfonate may be administered orally, or rectally as a retention enema. When the drug is in the bowel, potassium is exchanged for sodium; however, if hyperkalemia is severe, the patient may need dialysis to adequately decrease the potassium level.

139 C: When considering the stages of chronic kidney disease, a patient is considered in need of dialysis when the GFR falls to less than 15 mL/min/1.73 m². This is stage 5, and patients may also be considered for renal transplant if uremia is present. Some patients may live for many years with compromised kidney function while others may progress quite rapidly to stage 5, depending on many factors, including the patient's general condition, adherence to treatment, and age.

140. A: The primary treatment for chronic kidney disease-mineral and bone disorder (CKD-MBD) is decreasing hyperphosphatemia. Approaches include administration of phosphate binders, such as calcium acetate and calcium carbonate, and avoidance of the use of preparations with aluminum and magnesium. Secondary hyperparathyroidism should be treated with the activated form of vitamin D (because the kidneys can no longer activate it), using care to avoid hypercalcemia. Secondary hyperparathyroidism may also require cinacalcet, which mimics calcium.

141. C: Standards that cover medical devices used for dialysis, such as dialyzers and blood tubing, are set by the Food and Drug Administration (FDA). The FDA publishes *Quality Assurance Guidelines for Hemodialysis Devices* to provide guidance to hemodialysis units and centers and to outline the steps to quality assurance. The FDA has also published a draft guidance for implanted blood access devices, including subcutaneous catheters. Hemodialysis providers must report any problems with the medical devices in use and report all adverse events.

142. A: If a patient with uremia passes urine that is foamy or bubbly, this probably represents protein in the urine resulting from changes in the glomeruli that allow proteins to pass into the urine. With proteinuria, patients may also begin to exhibit generalized edema. Changes in urinary patterns are indicative of kidney failure. Patients may also experience more frequent urination and nocturia. The urine may contain blood. Urine may appear more concentrated or less concentrated.

143. B: If imaging shows that the kidneys have atrophied to about one-fifth the normal size, the most likely diagnosis is chronic glomerulonephritis. As the kidneys are damaged, the kidney tissue is replaced with fibrous tissue and the cortex layer of the kidney shrinks to 1 to 2 mm. The kidney surface becomes very irregular because of scar tissue. While patients may exhibit no symptoms until kidneys are severely damaged, some patients are diagnosed when they develop hypertension and elevated BUN and serum creatinine.

144. C: Patients are at increased risk of mortality when predialytic albumin levels fall to less than 4 g/dL with increased risk of morbidity with levels less than 3 g/dL. Albumin levels should be monitored before dialysis sessions at least every 3 months because the albumin level is an indicator of a patient's overall nutritional status. If the level is below normal, the cause should be identified and corrected as soon as possible.

145. A: Treatment for nephrotic syndrome usually includes diuretics to reduce edema, lipid-lowering agents to decrease hyperlipidemia and slow atherosclerosis, and ACE inhibitors to

reduce proteinuria. ARBs may also be used because they have similar protein-reducing effects. ACE inhibitors cause the efferent arterioles of the glomeruli to relax, reducing pressure within the glomeruli so that less protein is pushed into the urine. Commonly used ACE inhibitors for control of proteinuria include enalapril and captopril.

146. A: Glomerular filtration in which fluids and solutes are filtered from the blood is the first step in urine production, but reabsorption begins in the proximal convoluted tubule, which resorbs sodium, potassium, chloride, urea, glucose, and amino acid. Further reabsorption of electrolytes occurs in the loop of Henle, distal tubule, and collecting duct. The 3 processes involved in urine production are glomerular filtration, tubular reabsorption, and tubular secretion, which allows the body to reduce the concentration of substances in the blood, such as potassium or drugs.

147. C: If an older adult fractures a hip and lies immobile for long periods of time, the patient may develop muscle trauma and rhabdomyolysis, which can lead to kidney failure because of the release of creatinine and myoglobin from the damaged tissue. Because the patient was immobile, the cell membrane is damaged, allowing sodium and water to fill muscle cells. Neutrophils enter the edematous tissue and cause an inflammatory response and nephrotoxicity. The typical triad of symptoms includes muscle weakness, muscle pain, and dark urine. The urine becomes red-brown in color from leakage of myoglobin from the muscle cells.

148. D: The patient exhibits a number of signs and symptoms of uremia. Both diabetes and hypertension are risk factors, and increasing edema, nausea and vomiting, lethargy, and itching are common findings associated with uremia. The patient's blood pressure is uncontrolled on admission. The patient's laboratory results show signs of kidney failure, including hyperkalemia and hyperphosphatemia, as well as elevated BUN, serum creatinine, and parathyroid hormone. Additionally, the patient is anemic with a low hemoglobin and hematocrit.

149. C: For most patients on CAPD, glucose present in dialysate adds about 500 calories each day, so patients are at risk of increased weight gain. Patients should monitor their diet carefully, and dry weight should be routinely reassessed to determine if patients' weight gain is from fluid retention or increased fat stores. Because of the calories absorbed from dialysate, patients on peritoneal dialysis generally require a lower calorie/kg (30 to 35) than patients on HD.

150. B: The surface area of the peritoneal cavity, which lines the peritoneal cavity, in an adult is typically 1 to 2 m^2. The peritoneum comprises the visceral peritoneum (the lining of the gut and other viscera), which makes up about 80% of the total peritoneal surface area, and the parietal perineum (lining the abdominal cavity), which is the most important for peritoneal dialysis. The total blood flow in the peritoneum is estimated at 50 to 100 mL/min.

Section Description: Davis Case Questions

151. B: A catheter should be implanted about 2 weeks prior to a patient beginning peritoneal dialysis. At one time, even if a patient elected peritoneal dialysis, a backup AV fistula was created in case the PD was not effective or the patient decided to switch to hemodialysis, but this is no longer recommended. Sometimes a peritoneal catheter is placed temporarily when a patient is going to have hemodialysis if the need for dialysis is urgent.

152. A: When teaching a patient about peritoneal dialysis, the nurse should advise the patient that one advantage to peritoneal dialysis over hemodialysis is fewer restrictions in fluids and sodium. Fluid restriction is less stringent because of the more frequent dialysis, which removes excess fluid. Also, water passes through the peritoneal membrane more readily than through dialyzer membranes, increasing fluid loss. While hemodialysis patients must generally limit sodium intakes to 2 to 3 g daily, patients on peritoneal dialysis usually can have intake of 2 to 4 g daily.

153. A: Obesity is often a contraindication for peritoneal dialysis. Other contraindications include older adulthood and lack of social support, such as family members who can assist. Patients with ostomies or ventriculoperitoneal shunts are also usually advised against peritoneal dialysis. Indications for peritoneal dialysis include cardiovascular disease, younger age, adherence to treatment regimen, and adequate social support. The choice of peritoneal dialysis as opposed to hemodialysis should be made on an individual basis, considering many factors.

Section Description: Nguyen Case Questions

154. A: If a 58-year-old patient with type 2 diabetes and ESKD has been treated with hemodialysis for 2 years and develops numerous painful firm brown nodules on both lower legs with some nodules eroding and becoming necrotic, as well as mottled skin and decreased sensation, the most likely cause is calcific uremic arteriolopathy (CUA). CUA is a life-threatening disorder associated with kidney failure in which arterioles become calcified and result in necrosis of the tissue. It is more common in patients with diabetic comorbidity, and incidence is higher in females than males.

155. D: The treatment that is most commonly used to treat CUA is IV sodium thiosulfate. Biopsies carry a high risk of mortality but may help to guide treatment; surgical debridement is contraindicated. Corticosteroids and immunosuppressive agents may worsen the condition. Some studies have indicated that patients on PD seem to be at higher risk than those on HD, perhaps because phosphate levels tend to be higher with PD. Secondary hyperparathyroidism is also an increased risk factor because of resultant hyperphosphatemia.

Section Description: Bell Case Questions

156. B: Hypovolemia is a primary cause of muscle cramping during hemodialysis. Other common causes include hypotension, high ultrafiltration rate, and low-sodium dialysis solution. Muscle cramps occur when the muscles do not receive adequate perfusion because of vasoconstriction, so cramping frequently occurs with hypotension. Cramping is most likely to occur during the first month a patient receives hemodialysis. Both hypomagnesemia and hypocalcemia may precipitate muscle cramping.

157. D: If a patient on hemodialysis says that he is unable to work or care for his family and is increasingly sedentary because of severe episodes of fatigue, the most important intervention is to assess for causes of fatigue to determine if treatment may reduce the fatigue and allow the patient to function more normally. Fatigue is a very common effect of chronic kidney disease, occurring in over 60% of patients. Fatigue may be associated with hyperkalemia and anemia.

158. C: When documenting observations about a patient, the most appropriate description is, "Patient is sighing and rubbing hands together," because this is an objective observation. In documenting, the nurse should avoid subjective descriptions, such as "nervous and upset," "appears in a very good mood," and uncooperative and belligerent," because these descriptions are based on opinion and may be interpreted differently by others. In documenting, the nurse should describe what the patient is actually doing or saying.

159. C: If the patient has developed a small aneurysm and asks the nurse to cannulate the aneurysm for the hemodialysis treatment because another patient told him that it would be less painful than cannulation of the fistula, the best response is to advise the patient that cannulating an aneurysm may result in rupture. An aneurysm is a weak ballooning area of the vessel, and if it ruptures the patient could rapidly exsanguinate.

Section Description: Independent Questions, Group 5

160. C: The primary advantage of using a Y-set with preattached double bag system rather than a straight set for peritoneal dialysis is decreased incidence of peritonitis. This system, like the standard Y-set, also requires a flush-before-fill step, but the purpose is only to flush out air; bacteria is not likely to invade the system since there is no connection between the transfer set and the solution bag. This system is the most commonly used and is easier to use than other systems.

161. D: If a patient undergoing peritoneal dialysis and recovering from *Staphylococcus aureus* peritonitis is found to be a nasal carrier of *Staph*, the most commonly used prophylaxis is mupirocin cream intranasally twice daily for 5 days ever 4 weeks. An alternative treatment is oral rifampin 300 mg twice daily for 5 days every 3 months. If patients who are nasal carriers are not treated for the nasal infection, they are at high risk for recurrent peritonitis. Repeated cultures should be done to ensure that the nasal infection is controlled

162. B: When teaching a patient about peritoneal dialysis and dwell times, the patient should understand that the minimum dwell time necessary for adequate removal of wastes is usually about 2 hours. Most people use dwell times of 4 to 6 hours. Dwell times and the number of exchanges may vary depending on whether the patient is using CAPD, which requires no machine, or APD, which uses a machine to automatically cycle between dwell and drain, usually during the night.

163. D: A risk factor for development of hernia in patients undergoing peritoneal dialysis is obesity because of the stress obesity places on the musculature. Other risk factors include sitting position during dwells and use of large volumes of dialysate. Patients who have undergone recent abdominal surgery are also at increased risk as are multiparous women. Isometric exercises may strain the muscles and result in hernias. The Valsalva maneuver, which occurs when a patient coughs or strains to defecate, may also increase risk of hernia.

164. B: If a patient has been experiencing recent weight gain without generalized edema but with protuberant abdomen and if the returns of dialysate are less than the instilled volume, the nurse should suspect an abdominal wall leak. The fluid builds up in the abdominal wall, resulting in weight gain, and the abdomen begins to distend, often asymmetrically (best

viewed with the patient in standing position). The abdomen itself may appear edematous with waistbands making a deep impression, for example.

165. B: Following insertion of a peritoneal catheter and beginning of peritoneal dialysis, if the nurse notes that the dressing over the site is damp, a glucose dipstick test should be done to help determine if the cause is pericatheter leak. If there is a pericatheter leak of dialysate, which is relatively high in glucose, the dipstick test should test strongly positive for glucose. The leak may be confirmed with contrast CT scan.

166. A: If a patient tests positive for a pericatheter leak, the most common treatment is to drain the abdomen and stop peritoneal dialysis for up to 48 hours because most leaks around the catheter will heal in a short period of time. If the leak persists, the patient may be placed on hemodialysis for a few days to allow more time for healing. If prolonged rest does not stop the leak, then the catheter may need to be removed and a catheter placed in another site.

167. C: Because sudden onset of shortness of breath with the first dwell is consistent with hydrothorax, the immediate response should be to stop the dialysis to prevent further fluid from entering the pleural cavity. The patient should be assisted into sitting position and oxygen administered if necessary. Hydrothorax almost always occurs on the right side, so respirations should be evaluated. If necessary, a thoracentesis may be done to remove fluid. If the fluid withdrawn has high glucose content, this may help to confirm the diagnosis.

168. A: If a patient on CAPD has severe unremitting lower back pain, the best solution may be changing to APD with no daytime dwell. Because of the increase in intraabdominal pressure that occurs with a dwell, the center of gravity shifts, and this can put added stress on the lumbar vertebrae and muscles of the lower back. While bedrest and analgesia may provide some temporary relief, the pain is likely to recur unless the patient is in supine position during dwell time, but this is not practical with CAPD.

169. B: Long-term peritoneal dialysis places the patient at increased risk of hypokalemia. Up to 30% of patients on peritoneal dialysis exhibit hypokalemia, although the reasons may vary. Some potassium may be lost in effluent, and patients may have diets with insufficient potassium. Patients usually receive oral potassium supplements as treatment because intraperitoneal administration increases the risk of contamination and peritonitis.
- Normal values: 3.5-5.5 mEq/L.
- Hypokalemia: <3.5 mEq/L. Critical value: <2.5 mEq/L.
- Hyperkalemia: >5.5 mEq/L. Critical value: >6.5 mEq/L.

170. D: If the nurse serves as case manager for a patient who lives at considerable distance from the nurse's office in a rural area, and the patient uses CAPD and manages fairly well but is anxious about being so far from medical help, the best method of keeping in touch with the patient and managing the patient's care is probably video chat, such as with Skype or FaceTime. Face-to-face consultation, even per video, is reassuring to a patient who is anxious and allows the nurse to see the patient's equipment and monitor the patient's procedures.

171. C: If a new occupational therapist has started working with the dialysis team but has a different approach than the previous therapist, as the supervisor, the nurse's primary concern should be assessing the quality of care that the occupational therapist provides.

Change is not necessarily a bad thing, but it may seem threatening to some team members. If the occupational therapist is providing good care, then the nurse must communicate this with team members and help the team to recognize the therapist's contributions.

172. B: When a patient is being discharged from the hospital and will be referred to a home health agency for assistance with peritoneal dialysis, the best method to ensure that the patient understands the discharge plan is to telephone the patient after discharge to discuss the discharge plan. Patients are often confused about discharge plans and anxious about returning home, so a telephone call the day after discharge is often welcome and ensures the patient understands and follows through with the discharge plan.

173. A: If a hemodialysis patient routinely experiences hypotensive episodes near the end of a session and experiences malaise, muscle cramps, and dizziness after dialysis, the most likely cause is that the dry weight is set too low. If these symptoms occur, then the patient's dry weight may need to be adjusted. If the dry weight, the optimal post-dialysis weight, is set too high, the patient may experience fluid overload after dialysis, resulting in peripheral edema and/or pulmonary edema with subsequent ingestion of fluids.

174. D: Patients undergoing home hemodialysis are required to have a telephone within arm's reach while undergoing dialysis so that they can readily call for help if needed. In some cases, a landline is preferred over a cell phone because it is not dependent on being charged; however, some patients may feel more secure to have both a landline and a cell phone available. The 9-1-1 emergency number should be programmed into the telephones for ease of use.

175. C: A dopamine precursor, such as levodopa, is generally considered the medication of choice for restless legs syndrome (RLS), although benzodiazepines are also used. RLS is very common among patients with end-stage kidney disease. There is no objective test to diagnose RLS so diagnosis depends on patient report of symptoms, which are typically an irritating sensation in the legs and feet that is relieved only by movement. RLS occurs during periods when the patient is at rest, usually prior to the patient's usual bedtime.

Practice Test #2

Practice Questions

Section Description: Adler Case Questions (Questions 1–7)

Joseph Adler is a 38-year-old male with diabetes mellitus who has been on hemodialysis for the past 2 years. Mr. Adler's partner states that he has been increasingly withdrawn and disinterested, sleeping most of the day.

1. Mr. Adler is started on an SSRI (fluoxetine 20 mg daily) for treatment of depression. After two weeks, the patient reports no improvement. The patient should be advised that
    a. a different SSRI may be needed.
    b. SSRIs may be ineffective for the patient.
    c. four to six weeks are needed to evaluate response.
    d. the patient may respond better to other types of therapy.

2. If the patient continues to have persistent episodes of depression despite taking an SSRI for 3 months, which of the following non-pharmaceutical therapies may best help the patient to cope with the depression?
    a. Psychoanalysis.
    b. Cognitive behavioral therapy.
    c. Group therapy.
    d. Electroconvulsive therapy.

3. If one hemodialysis patient reacts to a complication with little apparent stress and copes well and another patient, such as Mr. Adler, reacts to the same complication with severe stress and anxiety and copes poorly, the difference may lie in the patients'
    a. sense of belonging.
    b. self-efficacy.
    c. resilience.
    d. hardiness.

4. Mr. Adler has recently begun missing treatments and failing to take prescribed medications, despite the adverse physical response. When queried, the patient appears cheerful and insists that he is fine but "busy" and "forgot" about the treatments. The nurse should consider
    a. suicidal ideation.
    b. dementia.
    c. an electrolyte imbalance.
    d. anxiety.

5. Mr. Adler states that one of his primary worries is that he is no longer able to work full time but is not eligible for Medicaid. The patient is concerned that he cannot afford to pay for his insurance. The organization that may provide financial assistance is the
    a. American Association of Kidney Patients.
    b. National Organization for Renal Disease.
    c. National Kidney Foundation.
    d. American Kidney Fund.

6. When considering a hemodialysis patient's socioeconomic status, the three factors to focus on are
    a. age, income, and education.
    b. residence, income, and race.
    c. income, education, and occupation.
    d. age, occupation, and income.

7. Mr. Adler's depression seems to improve over time, although the patient continues to have multiple problems. Additionally, he brings a dog to a clinic appointment with him without explanation. If the staff is unsure if the dog is a service animal, a question that is legally permitted is
    a. "What kind of disability do you have that requires a service animal?"
    b. "Do you have proof that this animal is certified?"
    c. "What jobs has the dog been trained to perform for you?"
    d. "Can you ask the dog to demonstrate carrying out a task?"

Section Description: Patel Case Questions (Questions 8-9)

Anita Patel is a 46-year-old woman who undergoes CAPD following kidney failure associated with chronic glomerulonephritis.

8. Ms. Patel has developed a pericatheter mass. The most common method to differentiate a hernia from a hematoma or seroma is to
    a. have the patient stand and bear down.
    b. evaluate through auscultation and palpation.
    c. examine with a CT scan.
    d. examine with an ultrasound.

9. Once it is determined that Ms. Patel has a hernia, the patient is scheduled for contrast-associated CT. The patient has 2 L of dialysate containing 100 mL of contrast material (Omnipaque 300) instilled into the peritoneal cavity. After instillation, the patient should
    a. immediately have the CT without any wait time.
    b. walk about or remain active for 2 hours and then have the CT.
    c. carry out normal routines for 5 hours and then have the CT.
    d. lie in the supine position for 2 hours and then have the CT.

Section Description: Williams Case Questions (Questions 10–12)

Sadie Williams is a 52-year-old female with chronic kidney disease resulting from hypertension and diabetes mellitus, type 1.

10. Ms. Williams complains of frequent nausea and a bad taste in her mouth and states that her spouse reports that her breath increasingly has an "ammonia" or "urine" smell. The most likely cause is
    a. dental caries.
    b. diabetic ketoacidosis.
    c. uremic fetor.
    d. gingivitis.

11. Although the patient's control of her glucose levels had been poor, she reports that her glycemic control has improved in recent weeks, although she has had recent episodes of hypoglycemia. The most likely reason for this is
    a. inadequate diet.
    b. hyperinsulinism.
    c. hypoinsulinism.
    d. diabetic ketoacidosis.

12. The patient complains of increasing weakness and fatigue, resulting in difficulty in carrying out activities of daily living, such as cooking, cleaning, and even dressing; and this is causing her frustration and anxiety. The most valuable resource for this patient is likely a(n)
    a. housekeeping service.
    b. physical therapist.
    c. psychiatrist.
    d. occupational therapist.

Section Description: Clark Case Questions (Questions 13-16)

Josh Clark is a 40-year-old HIV-positive patient utilizing hemodialysis for end-stage kidney disease.

13. Mr. Clark often experiences intradialytic hypotension. Which of the following preventive measures is usually the best approach for patients who routinely experience intradialytic hypotension because of volume-related problems associated with large intradialytic weight gain?
    a. Increasing the patient's dry weight.
    b. Extending weekly dialysis time.
    c. Increasing restriction of fluid intake .
    d. Increasing restriction of sodium intake.

14. If Mr. Clark's predialytic serum total cholesterol level falls to <150 mg/dL, this probably represents
    a. an optimal cholesterol level.
    b. excessive statin dosage.
    c. poor nutritional status.
    d. incorrect dialysate.

15. If Mr. Clark has persistent headaches during dialysis, the medication usually given to manage headaches is
    a. aspirin.
    b. NSAIDs.
    c. hydrocodone.
    d. acetaminophen.

16. During Mr. Clark's hemodialysis session, a low-pressure alarm for venous pressure sounds. This could indicate
    a. infiltration of the venous needle.
    b. a clotted dialyzer.
    c. clotting in the access.
    d. a poorly functioning central catheter.

Section Description: Johnson Case Questions (Questions 17 -- 21)

Grace Johnson is a 58-year-old female with diabetes mellitus, type 1 who is undergoing hemodialysis. The patient has had problems tolerating hemodialysis with numerous complications.

17. Ms. Johnson complains of severe muscle pain and stiffness. Medications include calcitriol 0.25 mg daily, atorvastatin 20 mg daily, insulin glargine 26 units twice daily, regular insulin per sliding scale as needed before meals and at bedtime, and furosemide 20 mg daily. Which of these medications is most likely the cause of the muscle pain?
    a. Atorvastatin.
    b. Calcitriol.
    c. Furosemide.
    d. Insulin glargine.

18. Ms. Johnson should be taught to monitor bowel function and to avoid constipation because constipation increases risk of:
    a. hypercalcemia.
    b. hypokalemia.
    c. hyperkalemia.
    d. hyperphosphatemia.

19. Ms. Johnson has not responded well to an erythropoiesis stimulating agent (ESA). Which of the following treatments is indicated specifically for hemodialysis patients with epoetin-resistant anemia?
    a. Iron infusion.
    b. L-carnitine.
    c. RBC transfusion.
    d. Oral ferrous sulfate.

20. During hemodialysis, Ms. Johnson, who is lying in the supine position, complains of chest pain, begins coughing, and shows evidence of cyanosis of the distal extremities and lips. The nurse should suspect that the patient has
    a. anaphylaxis.
    b. a myocardial infarction.
    c. disequilibrium syndrome.
    d. an air embolism.

21. To prevent further complications, the nurse should immediately
    a. clamp the venous line and stop the blood pump.
    b. provide nasal oxygen at 4 L/min.
    c. increase the blood flow rate and the dialysate flow rate.
    d. administer a saline bolus to the patient.

22. In response to these symptoms, the patient should be positioned
    a. upright at 90°.
    b. in the semi-Fowler's position.
    c. Trendelenburg on the left side or flat supine.
    d. Trendelenburg on the right side.

Section Description: Kim Case Questions (Questions 23–30)

Janine Kim is a 30-year-old female whose left kidney was removed at age 25, but now her right kidney is failing. Ms. Kim is preparing for hemodialysis and will have an AV fistula created.

23. When evaluating Ms. Kim in preparation for creation of a fistula, the blood pressure difference between the arms should be less than
    a. 5 mm Hg.
    b. 10 mm Hg.
    c. 15 mm Hg.
    d. 20 mm Hg.

24. When conducting the Allen test to assess circulation of the radial and ulnar arteries, arterial insufficiency is indicated when the blanching persists for
    a. ≥2 seconds.
    b. ≥3 seconds.
    c. ≥4 seconds.
    d. ≥5 seconds.

25. For preoperative assessment of vessels, Doppler ultrasonography is often done under regional anesthesia of the arm because
    a. it is a painful procedure.
    b. anesthesia causes the veins to dilate.
    c. anesthesia causes the veins to constrict.
    d. the patient must hold completely still.

26. Following a period of maturation after the creation of an AV fistula, what diameter of the AV fistula is considered necessary before the fistula can be used for hemodialysis?
   a. 3 mm.
   b. 6 mm.
   c. 1 cm.
   d. 1.5 cm.

27. When auscultating Ms. Kim's AV fistula to listen for the bruit, if the nurse notes the bruit is very high pitched. This may indicate
   a. normal functioning.
   b. collateral circulation.
   c. stenosis.
   d. inadequate anastomosis.

28. Ms. Kim asks about using the buttonhole technique for cannulation. When using the buttonhole technique for vascular access for hemodialysis, the needles are placed
   a. in the same sites in a graft.
   b. in rotating sites in a graft.
   c. in rotating sites in a fistula.
   d. in the same sites in a fistula.

29. When teaching Ms. Kim about inserting a needle for hemodialysis, which of the following should the patient understand increases the risk of infiltration?
   a. Rotating the needle 180 degrees.
   b. Flushing the needle with NS after insertion.
   c. Leveling the needle to the surface of the skin to advance.
   d. Using a wet needle for insertion.

30. Following formation of an AV fistula and beginning of hemodialysis, the nurse notes that Ms. Kim's nail beds and skin on the hand below the fistula are cyanotic during hemodialysis, and the patient complains of pain in the hand. This is likely an indication of
   a. steal syndrome.
   b. stenosis.
   c. aneurysm.
   d. infection.

Section Description: Independent Questions, Group 1 (Questions 31-51)

31. The permeability of a dialyzer membrane to water is indicated by its
   a. transmembrane pressure.
   b. osmotic ultrafiltration.
   c. diffusion pressure.
   d. ultrafiltration coefficient.

32. If a dialyzer is to be reprocessed in 3 hours, the dialyzer must be
   a. heated to body temperature (37 °C).
   b. frozen.
   c. maintained at room temperature.
   d. refrigerated.

33. What color is arterial blood tubing for hemodialysis most often color-coded?
   a. Red.
   b. Blue.
   c. Green.
   d. Yellow.

34. During hemodialysis, how much blood is usually outside of a patient's body at one time?
   a. 50 to 100 mL.
   b. 100 to 250 mL.
   c. 250 to 400 mL.
   d. 400 to 500 mL.

35. A hemodialysis center has set up a surveillance system to monitor bloodstream infections (BSIs). Once this event has been chosen for monitoring, what should be determined next?
   a. Methods of data collection.
   b. Methods of data analysis.
   c. Data elements for collection.
   d. Time period for observation.

36. For patients on oral iron, in order to increase absorption, patients should be advised to
   a. take the supplement with dairy products, such as milk.
   b. take enteric-coated preparations of the supplement.
   c. take the supplement on an empty stomach.
   d. take the supplement with phosphate binders.

37. According to the NHSN Dialysis Event Surveillance guide, the standardized infection ratio (SIR) is calculated based on the
   a. number of bloodstream infections (BSIs) observed in a facility.
   b. number of observed BSIs divided by the number of at-risk patients.
   c. number of predicted BSIs divided by the number of observed BSIs.
   d. number of observed BSIs divided by the number of predicted BSIs.

38. Which of the following molecules has the highest molecular weight?
   a. Creatinine.
   b. Urea.
   c. Calcium.
   d. Albumin.

39. Backwashing to free residue from sediment filters in the water system should be done at least
   a. every 8 hours.
   b. one time daily.
   c. every 4 hours.
   d. one time weekly.

40. If the usual dose of potassium in dialysate is 2.0 mM, what is the usual dose for a patient who is taking digitalis?
    a. 1.0 mM.
    b. 2.0 mM.
    c. 3.0 mM.
    d. 4.0 mM.

41. The physician has prescribed midodrine 10 mg for a patient to take 2 hours prior to hemodialysis. The most likely reason for this medication is to prevent intradialytic
    a. hypotension.
    b. hypertension.
    c. muscle cramps.
    d. nausea and vomiting.

42. In order to reuse dialyzers, the dialysis center must follow standards developed by the
    a. FDA.
    b. CMS.
    c. AAMI.
    d. OSHA.

43. Prior to using a reprocessed dialyzer, a recirculating rinse with NS should be completed with recirculating flow rate through the blood compartment and the dialysate compartment of at least
    a. 200 mL/min for BFR and 200mL/min for DFR.
    b. 200 mL/min for BFR and 500 mL/min for DFR.
    c. 500 mL/min for BFR and 200 mL/min for DFR.
    d. 500 mL/min for BFR and 500 mL/min for DFR.

44. When influencing others to continuously improve practice, the nurse should recognize that the first step in the change process is to
    a. believe in the possibility of change.
    b. decide to bring about change.
    c. take action to bring about change.
    d. understand the results of change.

45. As a leader of the interdisciplinary team, the nurse notes that a new team member is less productive than other team members and is often late finishing work. The best response is to
    a. remind the entire team of their responsibilities.
    b. speak directly with the team member about the observations.
    c. report the team member to a supervisor.
    d. give the team member a negative evaluation.

46. With the formula for urea kinetic modeling (UKM), the "K" in the Kt/V formula stands for
    a. duration of dialysis in minutes.
    b. mL of fluid in the patient's body.
    c. urea clearance (mL/min) plus residual urinary output.
    d. urea clearance (mL/min).

47. During peritoneal dialysis, the concentration gradient of a substance, such as urea
    a. decreases.
    b. increases.
    c. remains consistent.
    d. varies widely.

48. When considering interdisciplinary communication, which of the following is an example of collegial communication?
    a. The nurse reports on the patient's condition in a team meeting.
    b. The nurse responds to a patient's questions about occupational therapy.
    c. The nurse chats about vacation plans with the physical therapist over lunch.
    d. The nurse provides one-on-one instruction to a patient regarding wound care.

49. What is the purpose of the peritoneal equilibration test?
    a. Determine the amount of glucose absorbed from dialysate and the amount of urea and creatinine filtered into the dialysate in a 4-hour dwell.
    b. Determine the patient's serum urea and serum creatinine after a 4-hour dwell is drained.
    c. Determine the amount of urea in a 24-hour collection of drained dialysate compared to the amount of urea in the blood.
    d. Determine the amount of residual glucose that remains in the dialysate after a 4-hour dwell is drained.

50. Glucose in dialysate must be heat sterilized at a low pH in order to
    a. decrease generation of glucose degradation products.
    b. increase generation of glucose degradation products.
    c. prevent crystallization in the dialysate.
    d. prevent the dialysate from becoming cloudy.

51. The primary purpose of using an amino-based dialysate solution is for
    a. increased ultrafiltration.
    b. decreased ultrafiltration.
    c. electrolyte imbalance.
    d. nutritional supplementation.

Section Description: Walker Case Questions (Questions 52–53)

Denise Walker, a 62-year-old female on hemodialysis complains of persistent itching during hemodialysis.

52. If Ms. Walker's itching persists and the patient's Kt/V is 1.1, the first dialysis adjustment should be to
    a. decrease Kt/V to <1.0.
    b. increase Kt/V to >1.1.
    c. increase Kt/V to >1.2.
    d. increase Kt/V to >1.5.

53. If adjusting Ms. Walker's Kt/V and changing dialyzers do not relieve itching, the intervention most indicated is
   a. gabapentin.
   b. moisturizers/oil bath.
   c. tacrolimus ointment.
   d. UBV phototherapy.

Section Description: Chang Case Questions (Questions 54–61)

Tom Chang is a 65-year-old male patient with chronic kidney disease resulting from poorly controlled diabetes mellitus, type 2, and hypertension. Mr. Chang is aware that he will eventually need renal replacement therapy and is considering his options.

54. For a patient with chronic kidney disease, at what GFR should education about the different options for renal replacement therapy generally begin?
   a. ≤50 mL/min/1.73 m²
   b. ≤40 mL/min/1.73 m²
   c. ≤30 mL/min/1.73 m²
   d. ≤20 mL/min/1.73 m²

55. When teaching a patient about hemodialysis, the best way to determine that the teaching plan is geared to the patient's educational ability is to
   a. routinely simplify instructions based on the patient's nonverbal cues.
   b. assess the patient's abilities through a written test.
   c. assess vocabulary level during conversations.
   d. ask the patient directly about educational background and preferred style of learning.

56. When discussing options, the nurse points out that a disadvantage of hemodialysis as compared to peritoneal dialysis is
   a. poor control of blood pressure.
   b. increased risk of hypertriglyceridemia.
   c. increased risk of malnutrition.
   d. increased incidence of back pain.

57. If Mr. Chang chooses hemodialysis, which of the following is would be a contraindication?
   a. Hemodynamic instability.
   b. Metabolic acidosis.
   c. Changes in mentation.
   d. Hyperkalemia.

58. When teaching a patient about hemodialysis, the patient should understand that the primary advantage of short daily hemodialysis (at least 5 to 6 times weekly) is
   a. improved serum albumin levels.
   b. better control of anemia.
   c. improved nutritional measures.
   d. reduced left ventricular hypertrophy.

59. Mr. Chang is concerned about the time needed for dialysis. How many hours of peritoneal dialysis are approximately equivalent to 6 to 8 hours of hemodialysis?
    a. 12 to 20.
    b. 20 to 36.
    c. 36 to 48.
    d. 48 to 56.

60. Mr. Chang is considering CAPD. Which of the following may be a contraindication to CAPD?
    a. History of cervical disk disease.
    b. History of diverticulitis.
    c. The patient is legally blind.
    d. The patient is deaf.

61. Mr. Chang reports that his wife developed shingles, and he wonders if he should get the herpes zoster (shingles) vaccination. Patients with kidney disease considering the herpes zoster (shingles) vaccination should be advised to
    a. avoid the vaccination.
    b. take 1 dose if age 60 or older.
    c. take the dose if on immunosuppressive therapy.
    d. take 3 doses if age 65 or older.

Section Description: Pham Case Questions (Questions 62–66)

> Tony Pham is a 28-year-old male with a history of urinary tract infections. He comes to the ED with complaints of gross hematuria and bilateral flank pain.

62. An ultrasound is conducted to evaluate the patient's kidneys. Which of the following findings on ultrasound is diagnostic of autosomal dominant polycystic disease?
    a. Two or more total cysts.
    b. Two or more cysts in each kidney.
    c. Four or more total cysts.
    d. Four or more cysts in each kidney.

63. The patient is most at risk for additional cysts in the
    a. intestines.
    b. pancreas
    c. spleen.
    d. liver.

64. The gross hematuria associated with autosomal dominant polycystic kidney disease most often results from
    a. rupture of a cyst into the renal pelvis.
    b. development of renal lithiasis.
    c. a urinary tract infection.
    d. an infected renal cyst.

65. Mr. Pham reports that he has had three episodes of kidney stones over the previous 2 years. What type of kidney stone is most likely to occur in a patient with autosomal dominant polycystic kidney disease?
   a. Struvite.
   b. Cystine.
   c. Calcium oxalate.
   d. Uric acid.

66. If Mr. Pham develops sudden onset of excruciating pain in the lower back, right flank, and lower right abdomen, the most likely cause is
   a. infection.
   b. ischemia.
   c. hepatic cysts.
   d. bleeding in a cyst.

Section Description: Jackson Case Questions (Questions 67–68)

Ralph Jackson is a 27-year-old male diagnosed with anti-glomerular membrane glomerulonephritis (Goodpasture syndrome).

67. Goodpasture syndrome is typically characterized by kidney failure and
   a. liver failure.
   b. pulmonary hemorrhage.
   c. pancreatitis.
   d. splenomegaly.

68. The primary treatments for anti-glomerular membrane glomerulonephritis (Goodpasture syndrome) include
   a. plasmapheresis and corticosteroids.
   b. blood transfusions and cyclosporine.
   c. plasmapheresis and IgG.
   d. IgG and corticosteroids.

Section Description: Independent Questions, Group 2 (Questions 69-89)

69. According to KDOQI guidelines, when administering hemodialysis to a patient, a facemask should be worn
   a. for all access connections.
   b. if the nurse has a cough.
   c. if the patient has a cough.
   d. to discontinue the hemodialysis.

70. If two patients in the hemodialysis center are afebrile with no complaints at the onset of hemodialysis but begin to have chills and each spikes a fewer within 45 to 60 minutes, the most likely cause is
   a. local infection.
   b. a pyrogenic reaction.
   c. dialysis disequilibrium syndrome.
   d. systemic infection.

71. When inserting needles into a PTFE graft for hemodialysis, how far apart should the needle tips be?
   a. At least 1.0 inch.
   b. At least 1.5 inches.
   c. At least 2.0 inches.
   d. At least 2.5 inches.

72. If a patient on hemodialysis exhibits a change in personality and demonstrates increasingly aggressive and threatening behavior, the best response is to
   a. advise the patient that the behavior is inappropriate.
   b. refer for psychiatric evaluation.
   c. discontinue treating the patient.
   d. enlist the help of family members.

73. An adolescent patient has carried out peritoneal dialysis for 3 years, but on turning 18, the patient refuses further dialysis, stating he doesn't believe he needs it, although he is willing to take medications. He has moved out of his parents home and into an apartment with three friends. The best response is to
   a. refer the patient to a psychiatrist.
   b. provide education and support to the patient.
   c. advise the parents to get a court order mandating treatment.
   d. advise the parents to cut off all support until the patient agrees to dialysis.

74. Peritoneal dialysate is rendered hyperosmolar with the addition of
   a. glucose.
   b. sodium.
   c. bicarbonate.
   d. chloride.

75. A patient who has been carrying out peritoneal dialysis for three years has recently been developing episodes of increasing dyspnea with treatment and is suspected of having a hydrothorax. The patient is to have radionuclide scanning with technetium. After the technetium is instilled into the peritoneal cavity, the patient should be advised to
   a. lie quietly in the supine position between scans.
   b. sit in a chair and lean forward.
   c. remain ambulatory.
   d. massage the abdomen.

76. When a catheter is inserted for peritoneal dialysis, the length of the subcutaneous tunnel is usually
   a. 2 to 3 cm.
   b. 3 to 5 cm.
   c. 5 to 10 cm.
   d. 10 to 15 cm.

77. Rigid non-cuffed catheters should be used for peritoneal dialysis for a maximum of
   a. 24 hours.
   b. 3 days.
   c. 5 days.
   d. 7 days.

78. During the initial preoperative assessment while planning for insertion of a peritoneal catheter, the surgeon carries out stencil-based mapping to determine the optimal placement for the catheter. During this initial assessment, what marking on the skin is commonly done?
   a. None.
   b. Incision marks.
   c. Exit site.
   d. Incision marks, exit site, and tunnel track.

79. The most common cause of impaired outflow with peritoneal dialysis is
   a. thrombus.
   b. fibrous strands.
   c. dislodgement.
   d. constipation.

80. If a peritoneal catheter is placed but not used immediately, it should be irrigated within
   a. 2 hours.
   b. 12 hours.
   c. 36 hours.
   d. 72 hours.

81. A patient receiving peritoneal dialysis complains of discomfort at the exit site. On examination, the nurse notes that the subcutaneous cuff has extruded. What initial intervention does the nurse expect?
   a. Reinsertion of the cuff to the proper position.
   b. Shaving of the cuff.
   c. Removing the catheter.
   d. Catheter splicing.

82. According to KDOQI guidelines, how frequently should Kt/V urea be measured in patients after initiating peritoneal dialysis?
   a. After 1 week and then every month.
   b. After 1 week and then every 2 months.
   c. After 1 month and then every 4 months.
   d. After 1 month and then every 6 months.

83. According to NKF-DOQI clinical practice guidelines, peritoneal dialysis should be initiated when the Kt/V urea falls below
   a. 1.5.
   b. 2.0.
   c. 3.0.
   d. 4.0.

84. A symptom that is most specific for depression in a patient with uremia is
   a. changing patterns of sleep with frequent insomnia.
   b. feeling tired and lethargic.
   c. repeatedly thinking about dying.
   d. exhibiting psychomotor agitation.

85. What is the best time to discuss advance directives with a patient who is diagnosed with kidney failure?
   a. Upon patient request.
   b. Early after diagnosis.
   c. At stage 4.
   d. After initial renal replacement therapy.

86. Which of the following may result in a false positive for a urine albumin dipstick result?
   a. Increased urine sodium.
   b. Specific gravity of less than 1.010.
   c. Acidic urine.
   d. Presence of blood.

87. The most common reason for resistance to therapy with an erythropoiesis-stimulating agent (ESA) is
   a. allergic response.
   b. hyperlipidemia.
   c. hyperparathyroidism.
   d. iron deficiency.

88. In order to slow the progression of chronic kidney disease in patients with chronic metabolic acidosis, sodium bicarbonate should be administered to maintain the serum bicarbonate level at
   a. 1.2 mmol/L.
   b. 2.2 mmol/L.
   c. 22 mmol/L.
   d. 220 mmol/L.

89. The primary difference between glomerular filtrate and plasma is that glomerular filtrate does not contain
   a. amino acids.
   b. glucose.
   c. sodium.
   d. proteins.

Section Description: Schwartz Case Questions (Questions 90–93)

Ben Schwartz is a 58-year-old male who has been undergoing CAPD for the past year.

90. Mr. Schwartz informs the nurse that he has increased overall dwell time to compensate for skipping peritoneal dialysis two days per week. The best response is to
   a. tell the patient to resume his previous schedule.
   b. reassure the patient that this new schedule is appropriate.
   c. recommend the patient switch to hemodialysis.
   d. re-educate the patient about peritoneal dialysis.

91. Mr. Schwartz also reports that he had previously been doing 5 exchanges per day with CAPD but now is doing only 2 per day but with much longer dwell times to compensate. The best information to provide the patient is that this practice
    a. will result in reabsorption of effluent.
    b. is acceptable.
    c. will increase removal of toxins.
    d. will result in dehydration.

92. Mr. Schwartz resumes his previous schedule for CAPD but a month later reports a change in his residual urinary output. Mr. Schwartz initially had approximately 400 mL of residual urine daily, but the volume has been decreasing. In response to this change in residual kidney function, the patient will most likely need
    a. no change in peritoneal dialysis.
    b. shorter dwell times or lower volumes of dialysate.
    c. longer dwell times or larger volumes of dialysate.
    d. dialysate with a lower concentration of glucose.

93. Mr. Schwartz complains frequently about quality of life issues because of his need for dialysis. Which of the following assessment tools is most appropriate to assess quality of life?
    a. Katz index.
    b. Mini-Cog.
    c. Beck inventory.
    d. SF-36.

Section Description: Locke Case Questions (Questions 94 – 98)

Mary Ellen Locke is a 23-year-old female who developed acute kidney injury and renal failure after repeated bouts of glomerulonephritis. She has recently started peritoneal dialysis, APD with long-daytime dwell.

94. Ms. Locke calls to report that she has noted a small amount of blood in the effluent. The first question to ask the patient is
    a. "Do you have any abdominal pain?"
    b. "Do you feel weak or dizzy?"
    c. "Is there bleeding about the catheter exit site?"
    d. "Are you menstruating?"

95. Ms. Locke is very concerned about appearance and wants to know how much abdominal distention she should expect during dwell times. The average waist size increases by how much with CAPD?
    a. 1 to 2 inches.
    b. 2 to 4 inches.
    c. 4 to 6 inches.
    d. 6 to 8 inches.

96. Ms. Locke complains of a constant sweet taste in the mouth. The reason for this is probably
   a. dental disease.
   b. development of diabetes mellitus.
   c. gastric reflux from increased abdominal pressure.
   d. absorption of glucose from dialysate.

97. Ms. Locke has been losing weight and is becoming malnourished because her appetite is very poor and she feels full or slightly nauseated when she tries to eat a large meal. The best initial solution is probably to
   a. eat immediately after draining the dialysate.
   b. switch to APD.
   c. take additional vitamin supplements.
   d. eat small, frequent meals.

98. Ms. Locke's effluent shows many fibrin strands and clots, which are interfering with outflow. The recommended treatment is to
   a. add heparin to the dialysate.
   b. irrigate the tube with normal saline.
   c. irrigate the tube with heparin.
   d. provide exchange with amino-acid solution.

Section Description: Independent Questions, Group 3 (Questions 99-117)

99. If a patient is undergoing hemodialysis and the nurse notes that a bloodline has separated and blood has pooled beneath the access site, the first intervention should be to
   a. clamp both sides of separated line.
   b. stop the blood pump.
   c. reconnect the separated line.
   d. apply pressure at the outflow vein.

100. If a pseudoaneurysm occurs in a fistula, the most likely cause is
   a. infection.
   b. improper rotation of needle sites.
   c. inadequate anastomosis.
   d. incorrect needle size.

101. A patient who has had severe recurrent episodes of gout has recently started hemodialysis. What effect should the patient expect related to episodes of gout?
   a. Episodes of gout will be less responsive to medication therapy.
   b. Episodes of gout will likely increase in frequency.
   c. Hemodialysis should have no effect on gout.
   d. Episodes of gout should decrease.

102. A diabetic patient with chronic kidney disease is rapidly deteriorating and is starting hemodialysis. The patient has taken high doses of insulin for many years. What effects are end-stage kidney disease and dialysis likely to have on insulin dosage?
    a. The insulin dosage will likely remain the same.
    b. The insulin dosage will likely need to be increased.
    c. The insulin dosage will likely need to be decreased.
    d. The insulin dosage may vary widely from one day to another.

103. A patient undergoing hemodialysis has been anemic for the last few months. When the patient comes to the hemodialysis center for treatment, the nurse reviews the patient's laboratory report and finds that the patient's hemoglobin has dropped to 6.2 and hematocrit 19.1. The nurse is unable to reach the nephrologist but leaves a message. The best initial action is to
    a. continue with the dialysis treatment.
    b. hold the dialysis treatment until the physician responds.
    c. advise the patient to skip the dialysis treatment and make an appointment with the physician.
    d. telephone an alternate physician, such as the patient's internist.

104. A 70-year-old patient has developed dialysis-associated pericarditis with pericardial effusion, but the effusion had remained stable at about 75 mL in size. The patient has frequent echocardiograms, and the latest shows that the pericardial effusion has almost doubled in size. At what volume is surgical drainage usually considered?
    a. >150 mL.
    b. >200 mL.
    c. >250 mL.
    d. >350 mL.

105: If a hemodialysis patient is experiencing severe anxiety, an appropriate medication is
    a. lorazepam.
    b. phenobarbitol.
    c. gabapentin.
    d. diazepam.

106. For a patient who has been treated for bacterial peritonitis with IP antibiotics, what changes in nutritional status may occur?
    a. Increase glucose may result in weight gain.
    b. Loss of protein may result in malnutrition.
    c. Loss of fat may result in weight loss.
    d. Nutritional status should not be affected.

107. A patient on CAPD plans to take a trip out of state and stay for a week in a hotel. What is the best advice to help the patient plan for the trip?
    a. Plan to pack and take all supplies on the plane.
    b. Arrange to have supplies sent to the destination 2 to 4 weeks before arrival.
    c. Arrange with a local supplier at the destination to supply dialysate.
    d. Arrange for temporary hemodialysis in a center at the destination.

108. A patient is switching from CAPD with a nighttime dwell to APD with a daytime dwell. What adjustment in the procedure is likely to result when receiving dialysis during sleep?
	a. Decreased volume of dialysate for nighttime dwells.
	b. Increased volume of dialysate for nighttime dwells.
	c. Fewer exchanges in a 24-hour period.
	d. More exchanges in a 24-hour period.

109. A patient on peritoneal dialysis has erythema about the exit site and purulent discharge, although the dialysate solution returns clear. While awaiting the results of culture and sensitivities, the patient is started on antibiotics. Which organism should always be covered by empiric therapy?
	a. *Staphylococcus aureus.*
	b. *Pseudomonas aeruginosa.*
	c. Streptococci.
	d. Diptheroids.

110. The primary advantage to the use of the post-dilution mode for hemodiafiltration is
	a. hemodilution.
	b. accommodation of suboptimal blood flow.
	c. high solute clearance of low to high molecular weight solutes.
	d. reduced viscosity and oncotic pressure.

111. A diabetic patient receiving acute hemodialysis is hyperglycemic with glucose level of 270 mg/dL. Which electrolyte imbalance is of primary concern for this patient?
	a. Hyponatremia.
	b. Hypernatremia.
	c. Hypokalemia.
	d. Hyperkalemia.

112. If a patient scheduled for acute hemodialysis has a serum sodium level of 132 mmol/L, the initial goal should be to maintain the serum sodium level at
	a. ≥ 130 mmol/L.
	b. ≥ 140 mmol/L.
	c. ≥ 150 mmol/L.
	d. ≥ 160 mmol/L.

113. A patient who is scheduled for acute hemodialysis is severely hyperkalemic with abnormalities noted on ECG, including depressed P waves, peaked T waves, and widening of the QRS complex. The patient feels severe weakness and appears lethargic. While awaiting hemodialysis, which of the following treatments is most appropriate?
	a. Sodium bicarbonate infusion.
	b. Insulin infusion.
	c. Normal saline infusion.
	d. Calcium chloride infusion.

114. A patient involved in a sudden deceleration automobile accident experienced a severe blunt injury to the abdomen and complains of severe abdominal pain and has hematuria. The preferred method of evaluating for renal trauma is
   a. IVP.
   b. CT scan.
   c. ultrasound.
   d. angiography.

115. In order to be a candidate for renal transplant, the patient's GFR usually must be
   a. ≤50 mL/min/1.73 m².
   b. ≤40 mL/min/1.73 m².
   c. ≤30 mL/min/1.73 m².
   d. ≤20 mL/min/1.73 m².

116. Which of the following is usually considered an absolute contraindication for kidney transplant?
   a. Lack of financial resources/insurance to cover costs.
   b. BMI >35.
   c. History of malignancy within the past 5 years.
   d. Hepatitis C infection.

117. When teaching a patient about kidney transplantation, the patient should understand that the average lifespan of a transplanted kidney is:
   a. 5 to 7 years.
   b. 7 to 10 years.
   c. 10 to 15 years.
   d. 15 to 20 years.

Section Description: Rivera Case Questions (Questions 118–123)

Salvador Rivera is a 68-year-old male with chronic kidney disease and diabetes mellitus, type 2.

118. Mr. Rivera has severe peripheral nephropathy, hypertension, and proteinuria. His cholesterol level is 240. His GFR is 58 mL/min/1.73². Mr. Rivera has been taking metformin, an ACE inhibitor, a statin, and a thiazide diuretic. The patient's latest serum creatinine is 1.7. Which medication is cause for concern?
   a. Statin.
   b. ACE inhibitor.
   c. Thiazide diuretic.
   d. Metformin.

119. If Mr. Rivera's LDL level is 142, the goal of statin therapy and diet should be to decrease the patient's LDL to at least
   a. <100 mg/dL.
   b. <90 mg/dL.
   c. <70 mg/dL.
   d. <60 mg/dL.

120. Mr. Rivera is scheduled for a serum creatinine test. Mr. Rivera should be counseled to avoid which of the following for 8 hours before a serum creatinine test?
    a. Strenuous exercise and red meat.
    b. Dairy products.
    c. A bath or shower.
    d. Anticoagulant drugs.

121. A patient is scheduled for an IVP. When instructing the patient about preparation for the procedure, the patient should be advised to expect which of the following?
    a. There is no special preparation.
    b. The patient will be NPO for 8 hours prior to the test only.
    c. The patient will have a bowel prep and will be NPO for 8 hours prior to the test.
    d. The patient will have a bowel prep only before the test.

122. Diabetic nephropathy results from damage to the
    a. glomeruli.
    b. renal artery.
    c. loops of Henle.
    d. proximal convoluted tubules.

123. When a patient is severely dehydrated and hypotensive, the hypertonic plasma that results
    a. stimulates the kidneys to secrete angiotensin.
    b. stimulates the parathyroid gland to release parathyroid hormone.
    c. stimulates the kidneys to release erythropoietin.
    d. stimulates the posterior pituitary to release ADH.

Section Description: Williamson Case Questions (Questions 124–126)

Carol Williamson is a 42-year-old female patient who presents with sudden onset of hematuria, fever of 39 °C, nausea, anorexia, severe left costovertebral angle pain, and tenderness in the left flank on palpation.

124. Based on these symptoms, the most likely diagnosis is
    a. acute glomerulonephritis.
    b. chronic glomerulonephritis.
    c. acute pyelonephritis.
    d. chronic pyelonephritis.

125. The physician orders a clean-catch urine for urinalysis and culture and sensitivities, a CBC, a dipstick leukocyte esterase test, and a nitrite production test. The purpose of the nitrite production test is to evaluate for the presence of
    a. purulent material in the urine.
    b. bacteria in the urine.
    c. viral particles in the urine.
    d. fungi in the urine.

126. Ms. Williamson is treated in the ED with a dose of parenteral ceftriaxone and discharged with a prescription for ciprofloxacin 500 mg twice daily. How many days should the patient expect to take the oral antibiotics if no complications arise?
   a. 7 days.
   b. 14 days.
   c. 21 days.
   d. 38 days.

Section Description: Anna Bukowski (Questions 127–128)

127. A 32-year-old female patient has developed fever, maculopapular rash, pyuria, and acute renal insufficiency, suggestive of acute interstitial nephritis. The most common cause for the development of acute interstitial nephritis is
   a. hypokalemia.
   b. Sjögren syndrome.
   c. systemic lupus erythematosus.
   d. drugs.

128. Which blood abnormality is a common finding with acute interstitial nephritis?
   a. Decreased hemoglobin.
   b. Increased eosinophils.
   c. Increased monocytes.
   d. Increased lymphocytes.

Section Description: Andre Robinson Case Questions (Questions 129–134)

Andre Robinson is a 76-year-old male with chronic kidney failure. He has begun to gain excessive weight, and blood tests indicate the patient is no longer adhering to his dietary restrictions.

129. Mr. Robinson admits that he understands his dietary needs but finds cooking too difficult and has been eating primarily foods delivered from a fast-food restaurant across the street from his apartment. The most useful response is probably to
   a. refer the patient to a Meals on Wheels program.
   b. refer the patient to the renal dietitian.
   c. recommend the patient to an occupational therapist.
   d. remind the patient of the importance of diet.

130. Mr. Robinson's sister reports that the patient is having fluctuating periods of inattention, disorientation, and general confusion. Which of the following tools is intended to assess the development of delirium in patients as opposed to other causes of altered mental status?
   a. MMSE.
   b. Mini-Cog.
   c. Palliative Performance Scale.
   d. Confusion Assessment Method.

131. The nurse assesses the patient's mental status. Which of the following tasks is appropriate to assess a patient's ability to concentrate?
   a. Naming the current president.
   b. Providing the patient's social security number.
   c. Stating the city and state of residence.
   d. Repeating the days of the week backward.

132. Mr. Robinson's condition deteriorates, and tests show he has almost reached stage 5 chronic kidney disease, but he is not a candidate for transplantation and the patient's prognosis, even with dialysis, is very poor because of multiple co-morbidities. The best solution is to
   a. carry out a hemodialysis trial.
   b. discuss prognosis and options with the patient.
   c. provide palliative care only.
   d. discuss options with family members.

133. Mr. Robinson's PTH levels are elevated. For a patient with non-dialytic chronic kidney disease and elevated levels of PTH, the KDIGO guidelines recommend treatment with
   a. vitamin D.
   b. calcium.
   c. prednisone.
   d. cinacalcet.

Section Description: Independent Questions, Group 4 (Questions 134-159)

134. The most important consideration for patients in their approaches to health beliefs and health practices is usually
   a. educational background.
   b. cultural background.
   c. individual factors.
   d. socioeconomic status.

135. Prior to beginning treatment for diabetes, the patient's Hgb A1C was greater than 10%. What is a realistic target goal Hgb A1C for this patient?
   a. <9%.
   b. <8%.
   c. <7%.
   d. <6%.

136. For a patient at stage 4 kidney disease considering options, the patient should understand that the best survival rate is associated with
   a. post-dialytic transplantation.
   b. pre-emptive transplantation.
   c. hemodialysis.
   d. peritoneal dialysis.

137. The three processes involved in the production of urine are
   a. glomerular filtration, hormonal stimulation, and tubular reabsorption.
   b. glomerular filtration, tubular reabsorption, tubular secretion.
   c. glomerular filtration, ultrafiltration, and tubular reabsorption.
   d. glomerular filtration, sodium regulation, and tubular reabsorption.

138. The normal ratio of BUN to creatinine is
   a. 10:1.
   b. 8:1.
   c. 4:1.
   d. 2:1.

139. If a patient with a Foley catheter requires a 24-hour urine collection for the creatinine clearance test, the proper procedure to collect the specimen is to
   a. collect the urine from the catheter bag at the end of 24 hours.
   b. place the catheter bag in a container of ice and collect urine every 8 hours.
   c. place the catheter bag in container of ice and collect urine every hour.
   d. collect the urine from the catheter bag every hour.

140. A hospitalized patient who is incontinent of urine has undergone a renal scan. What, if any, precaution is needed by the nurse following the procedure?
   a. Gloves should be worn while handling urine and changing soiled linens.
   b. Gown, gloves, and facemask should be used when handling urine and changing soiled linens.
   c. No precautions are needed.
   d. A Foley catheter should be placed to safely collect urine.

141. A patient with kidney failure is to be assessed for possible vesicoureteral reflux (VUR). The test most indicated to confirm VUR is a(n)
   a. MRI.
   b. IVP.
   c. voiding cystourethrogram.
   d. cystoscopy.

142. Following kidney transplantation, the patient requires medications not covered by his insurance drug plan, and the patient tells the nurse that he is concerned that he may have to sell his home to pay for the drugs. The best response is to
   a. reassure the patient that a solution will be found.
   b. refer the patient to a social worker.
   c. suggest the patient apply for disability.
   d. suggest the patient ask the physician about different medications.

143. A 38-year-old patient will soon require dialysis but lives 2 hours from a dialysis center. The patient wants to carry out home dialysis so she can continue working and avoid disrupting her daily activities but lives alone and has no one available to assist her. The best option for the patient is probably
   a. in-center nocturnal dialysis.
   b. home hemodialysis.
   c. CAPD.
   d. APD.

144. Which of the following HIV-infected groups is most at risk for development of HIV-associated nephropathy (HIVAN)?
    a. Caucasian males.
    b. African American males.
    c. Asian females.
    d. Caucasian females.

145. Which of the following infections is commonly associated with membranous nephropathy?
    a. Hepatitis A-related glomerulonephritis.
    b. Hepatitis B-related glomerulonephritis.
    c. Hepatitis C-related glomerulonephritis.
    d. HIV-associated nephropathy.

146. With chronic kidney failure, vascular calcification results from
    a. hyperphosphatemia.
    b. hypophosphatemia.
    c. hypercalcemia.
    d. hyperkalemia.

147. A patient's urine osmolality is 300 Osm/kg. This probably indicates
    a. a normal value.
    b. dehydration.
    c. early kidney disease.
    d. end-stage kidney disease.

148. How many grams of urea are usually produced and excreted in 24 hours?
    a. 5 to 10g.
    b. 20 to 30 g.
    c. 40 to 50 g.
    d. 60 to 70 g.

149. A positive Chvostek sign is associated with
    a. hyperkalemia.
    b. hypokalemia.
    c. hypercalcemia.
    d. hypocalcemia.

150. Antidiuretic hormone (ADH) is secreted in response to
    a. an increase in blood osmolality.
    b. a decrease in blood osmolality.
    c. release of aldosterone.
    d. increased angiotensin II levels.

151. The kidneys regulate the acid-base balance by (1) reabsorbing bicarbonate and (2)
    a. excreting acid.
    b. excreting protein.
    c. reabsorbing acid.
    d. reabsorbing protein.

152. The most common cause of secondary glomerular disease is
    a. HIV-associated nephropathy.
    b. sickle-cell nephropathy.
    c. diabetic nephropathy.
    d. collagen-vascular diseases.

153. The three most common cardiovascular complications associated with chronic kidney disease are (1) hypertension, (2) congestive heart failure, and (3)
    a. atrial fibrillation.
    b. heart block.
    c. ventricular tachycardia.
    d. pericarditis.

154. A 68-year-old female patient with chronic kidney disease has been ambulatory but has come to the last two physician visits in a wheelchair. When questioned, the patient states that she is able to walk but finds that she is increasingly weak and has little stamina, so she resorts to a wheelchair. The best response is probably to refer the patient to a(n)
    a. psychologist.
    b. occupational therapist.
    c. physical therapist.
    d. social worker.

155. If a patient with chronic kidney disease has started to make threats against a member of his family and states that he wants the person dead and plans to use a gun to kill the person, the responsibility is to
    a. refer the patient to a psychiatrist.
    b. maintain the patient's confidentiality.
    c. notify the police.
    d. warn the person to whom the threats are directed.

156. Infection with *Clostridium difficile* may lead to kidney failure primarily because of
    a. migration of bacteria into the kidney.
    b. bacteremia.
    c. dehydration.
    d. sepsis.

157. A patient with chronic kidney disease has developed increasing urinary incontinence. The patient's caregiver has requested that the patient have a Foley catheter inserted to make care easier. The primary reason that Foley catheters are avoided in patients is because of
    a. risk of infections.
    b. increased costs.
    c. risk of bladder perforation.
    d. risk of urethral trauma/ulcerations.

158. The primary coagulopathy associated with chronic kidney disease is
   a. thrombocytosis.
   b. factor II (prothrombin) deficiency.
   c. factor X deficiency.
   d. platelet dysfunction.

159. If normal intake of potassium is about 100 mEq (3900 mg) per day, what is the usual limit for potassium if a patient's GFR has fallen to 15 mL/min?
   a. <20 to 30 mEq/d.
   b. <40 to 50 mEq/d.
   c. <50 to 60 mEq/d
   d. <60 to 70 mEq/d.

Section Description: Brown Case Questions (Questions 160–162)
   James Brown, a 70-year-old male with chronic kidney disease, presents in the ED with signs of uremia, including anorexia, nausea, fatigue, altered mental status, and signs of pericarditis with pericardial friction rub.

160. Immediate acute hemodialysis is needed to prevent
   a. pulmonary emboli.
   b. atrial fibrillation.
   c. myocardial infarction.
   d. cardiac tamponade.

161. Mr. Brown's blood urea nitrogen level is 130 mg/dL. What should the initial target urea reduction be?
   a. <20%.
   b. <40%.
   c. <60%.
   d. <80%.

162. When a venous catheter is inserted into the femoral vein for acute hemodialysis, the tip of the catheter should extend to the
   a. inferior vena cava.
   b. superior vena cava.
   c. internal iliac vein.
   d. right atrium.

Section Description: Torres Case Questions (Questions 163–164)

   Ramona Torres is a 50-year old female who is admitted to the ED in acute distress. The patient reports having fever and dysuria for the past week.

163. Ms. Torres has developed sepsis as the result of a urinary tract infection, resulting in acute kidney injury (AKI) and the need for continuous veno-venous hemofiltration (CVVH). The maximum dose for dialysis is
   a. 15 mL/kg/hr.
   b. 25 mL/kg/hr.
   c. 35 mL/kg/hr.
   d. 45 mL/kg/hr.

164. Ms. Torres has a catheter placed in the right jugular vein. In order to avoid puncture of the carotid artery when a venous catheter for acute hemodialysis is placed in the right internal jugular vein of a patient with sepsis, the best preventive is
   a. anatomic landmark guidance.
   b. angiography.
   c. ultrasound.
   d. radiography.

Section Description: Whitlow Case Questions (Questions 165–167)

Alton Whitlow is a 66-year-old male who had a kidney transplantation because of kidney failure associated with diabetes and hypertension.

165. Ten months after kidney transplant, Mr. Whitlow develops severe hypertension and pulmonary edema as well as increasing signs of acute kidney injury with increasing serum creatinine. The surgeon suspects renal artery stenosis. The test that is most commonly used to confirm the diagnosis is
   a. angiography.
   b. CT scan.
   c. MR angiography.
   d. radiograph.

166. Which of the following is a risk factor for renal artery stenosis?
   a. Hepatitis B infection.
   b. Hepatitis C infection.
   c. Cytomegalovirus infection.
   d. Fungal infection.

167. After confirmation of the advanced renal artery stenosis, the treatment of choice is most often
   a. vasodilators.
   b. transluminal angioplasty with/without placement of stents.
   c. surgical revascularization.
   d. hemodialysis.

Section Description: Abramov Case Questions (Questions 168–172)
Natasha Abramov is a 44-year-old patient who has received a deceased donor kidney because of polycystic kidney disease.

168. Since Ms. Abramov has received a deceased donor kidney, what information about the donor can be shared with the recipient?
   a. General location, age, and gender.
   b. Age, gender, and race.
   c. Address, name, and age.
   d. Name, age, and gender.

169. Which of the patient's drugs is classified as an antiproliferative and is often used in maintenance therapy after kidney transplantation?
    a. Cyclosporine.
    b. Tacrolimus.
    c. Prednisone.
    d. Mycophenolate mofetil.

170. Two weeks after kidney transplantation, Ms. Abramov has experienced an increase in temperature and flu-like symptoms as well as weight gain of 2.5 kg in 48 hours with decreased urinary output and pain in the operative site. The patient is scheduled for a core biopsy to determine if she is experiencing rejection. What guidance is usually used for the core biopsy?
    a. Anatomic guidelines.
    b. CT scan.
    c. Ultrasound.
    d. Angiography.

171. If the patient is confirmed through renal biopsy as having acute rejection, which of the following initial treatments is usually indicated?
    a. Corticosteroids.
    b. OKT3.
    c. High-dose cyclosporine.
    d. High-dose tacrolimus.

172. If Ms. Abramov develops hand tremors, back and abdominal pain, somnolence, loss of memory, and dark urine as well as increased serum creatinine and BUN, the medication that is most likely responsible is
    a. mycophenolate mofetil.
    b. cyclosporine.
    c. tacrolimus.
    d. prednisone

Section Description: El-Amin Case Questions (Questions 173–175)

El-Amin is a 56-year-old male who has received a living donor kidney from his 48-year-old brother.

173. Mr. El-Amin received basiliximab perioperatively and tacrolimus and mycophenolate mofetil (MMF) as immunosuppressive therapy. The patient was placed on a corticosteroid for one week only. Early steroid withdrawal is most associated with which of the following complications?
    a. Hyperlipidemia.
    b. Mortality.
    c. Acute rejection.
    d. Graft loss.

174. With kidney transplantation, therapy with basiliximab is primarily used to
    a. prevent T-cell replication and organ rejection.
    b. potentiate the effects of other immunosuppressive agents.
    c. reduce the risk of post-operative infection.
    d. reduce the risk of post-operative renal stenosis.

175. Following hospital discharge a week after a kidney transplantation, the patient had been doing well but has sudden onset of fever of 38.8 °C, chills, tenderness about the incision, and headache. The urine appears cloudy. The most likely cause is
    a. acute rejection.
    b. infection.
    c. hyperacute rejection.
    d. delayed graft function.

Answers and Explanations

Section Description: Adler Case Questions

1. C: If a patient with ESKD and hemodialysis is started on an SSRI (fluoxetine 20 mg) daily for treatment for depression but shows no improvement after two weeks, the patient should be advised that four to six weeks are needed to evaluate response. Tricyclic antidepressants are associated with more adverse effects and are usually avoided. Depression adversely affects quality of life and increases the risk of both morbidity and mortality. Depression is common in patients with chronic kidney disease and is often exacerbated by hemodialysis.

2. B: If a patient on hemodialysis has persistent episodes of depression despite taking an SSRI, the non-pharmaceutical therapy that may best help the patient to cope is cognitive behavioral therapy. CBT helps patients to change the way they think about things and provides methods to help substitute positive thoughts for negative ones. Patients are taught to recognize automatic thoughts (cognitive distortions) such as all-or-nothing thinking, catastrophizing, "mind reading," and personalization. Treatment is usually relatively short term (5 to 20 sessions).

3. C: If one hemodialysis patient reacts to a complication with little apparent stress and copes well and another patient reacts to the same complication with severe stress and anxiety and copes poorly, the difference may lie in the patients' resilience. Resilience is the ability to respond to stressful situations in a healthy and productive manner. A high degree of resilience allows a patient to cope well. Resilience is often associated with a positive outlook, good family support, and spirituality.

4. A: If a patient on hemodialysis with a history of ongoing depression has recently begun missing treatments and failing to take prescribed medications, despite adverse physical response, and the patient appears cheerful and insists he is find but "busy" and "forgot" about the treatments, the nurse should consider suicidal ideation. When hemodialysis patients skip treatments and medications, they are putting their lives at risk, and this provides an easy method of suicide. Once patients have decided to commit suicide, they may sometimes appear to be in a better mood, even cheerful.

5. D: The American Kidney Fund provides financial assistance to patients on dialysis through a number of programs:
- Grants Management System (GMS): Patients can apply directly for grants.
- Health Insurance Premium Program (HIPP): Provides assistance with Medicare part B, Medigap, COBRA, and other insurance premiums.
- Safety Net Grants: Assists with treatment-related expenses that are not covered by insurance.
- Sanofi Renal/Genzyme Patient Assistance Programs: Provides Renvela® and IV formulations of Hectorol® for those with no prescription drug coverage.
- Prescription Drug Resources: Provides lists of drug companies with special programs and resources for those without prescription drug coverage.

6. C: When considering a patient's socioeconomic status, the three factors to focus on are income, education, and occupation. Income can influence the patient's access to healthcare, adequate housing, and nutritious foods. Patients with little income often have few of the options available to those with high income. Education may influence the patient's choices and understanding of disease. Occupation may affect the patient's ability to remain employed. For example, blue-collar workers may find it much harder to continue working because of physical limitations when compared to white-collar workers.

7. C: If a patient brings a dog to a clinic appointment and the staff is unsure if the dog is a service animal, a question that is legally permitted is "What jobs has the dog been trained to perform for you?" It is also legal to ask if the dog is needed because of a disability, but it is not legal to ask what the disability is, to ask for proof that the animal is certified or trained, or to have the animal demonstrate its skills.

Section Description: Patel Case Questions

8. D: If a patient has developed a pericatheter mass, the most common method to differentiate a hernia from a hematoma or seroma is through ultrasonography, which will show if the mass is fluid-filled. The ultrasound is relatively inexpensive and non-invasive. All different types of hernias (including ventral, pericatheter, umbilical, inguinal, and femoral hernia) are common with peritoneal dialysis, occurring in up to 20% of patients. Risk factors include use of high volume dialysate, sitting, carrying out the Valsalva maneuver, obesity, and multiparity.

9. B: If a patient is to have a contrast-associated CT to help demonstrate the extent of the hernia, then 2L of dialysate containing the contrast material (usually Omnipaque 300) is instilled into the peritoneal cavity. After the instillation, the patient should be advised to walk about or remain active for 2 hours because this helps move the dye about freely in the peritoneal cavity and into the hernia. The CT scan is not always necessary, depending on the site of the hernia. For example, the extent of an umbilical hernia may be quite evident on examination.

Section Description: Williams Case Questions

10. C: If a patient with stage 4 chronic kidney disease complains of frequent bad taste in the mouth and states that her breath increasingly has an "ammonia" or "urine" smell, the most likely cause is uremic fetor, which develops as chronic kidney disease progresses to stage 5, kidney failure. As excess urea in the body breaks down in the saliva, it produces ammonia, which gives off a urine-like odor.

11. B: If a patient with chronic kidney disease and type 1 diabetes mellitus reports that her glycemic control has improved in recent weeks although she has had recent episodes of hypoglycemia, the most likely reason is that the patient has developed hyperinsulinism, a common occurrence with kidney failure. The half-life of insulin is also prolonged, so patients are likely to require decreased doses of insulin (or in some cases, no insulin) and are at risk for hypoglycemia.

12. D: Because the patient's increasing weakness and fatigue have made it difficult to carry out activities of daily living, such as cooking, cleaning, and dressing, the best resource is probably an occupational therapist. The therapist can assess the patient in the home

environment and can determine whether modifications or assistive devices could help the patient to manage better and to remain as independent as possible. If the patient's frustration and anxiety persist, the patient may benefit from a psychiatrist or other therapist.

Section Description: Clark Case Questions

13. D: The preventive measure that is usually the best approach for patients who routinely experience intradialytic hypotension because of volume-related problems associated with large intradialytic weight gain is to increase restriction of sodium intake. Patients who experience intradialytic hypotension are at increased risk of poor outcomes. Blood pressure should generally be maintained at a systolic pressure of at least 90 mm Hg. Low predialytic blood pressure is often an indicator for intradialytic hypotension.

14. C: If a patient's predialytic serum total cholesterol level falls to <150 mg/dL, this probably represents poor nutritional status, usually associated with a low serum albumin level. Both poor nutrition and inflammation may result in lowered cholesterol levels. Patients who maintain their serum cholesterol between 200 and 250 mg/dL tend to have a lower risk of mortality, and levels of less than 150 mg/dl are associated with increased risk. There is some debate about the use of statins because of this, but patients on dialysis are also at high risk of cardiovascular disease.

15. D: If a patient has persistent headaches during dialysis, the medication usually given for their management is acetaminophen. Up to 70% of patients on dialysis complain of headaches, and dialysis may exacerbate migraines. Headaches may result from hypomagnesemia, although magnesium supplementation must be used with caution in patients with kidney failure. NSAIDs are usually avoided because of their nephrotoxic affects, and aspirin should be avoided with heparin use during dialysis.

16. B: If a low-pressure alarm for venous pressure sounds during hemodialysis, this could indicate a clotted dialyzer. Other causes of the low-pressure alarms include separation of the blood tubing from the venous needle or catheter, decreased blood flow rate, and blockage of the blood tubing before the monitoring site. A high-pressure alarm for venous pressure may indicate blockage of the blood tubing between the venous needle and the monitoring site, infiltration of the venous needle, poorly functioning central catheter, or access clotting.

Section Description: Johnson Case Questions

17. A: If a patient on hemodialysis complains of severe muscle pain and stiffness, the medication that is most likely the cause is atorvastatin, as statins are associated with myopathy. The extent of myopathy may vary widely and symptoms usually recede within 2 months of stopping the medication, although some patients may develop rhabdomyolysis and persistent muscle damage. The patient may tolerate a different statin, or non-statin agents may be used.

18. C: A patient on hemodialysis should be taught to monitor bowel function and to avoid constipation because constipation increases risk of hyperkalemia. With normal kidney function, only about 5 to 10% of the potassium load is excreted through the intestines because the kidneys excrete the rest, but with impaired kidney function, the intestines

increase excretion up to 25%. Thus, constipation directly impacts potassium excretion, although hyperkalemia usually involves constipation coupled with excessive potassium intake.

19. B: L-carnitine, a naturally produced amino acid, is indicated specifically for hemodialysis patients with epoetin-resistant anemia. Patients on hemodialysis frequently are deficient in L-carnitine because of both poor nutritional intake and loss during dialysis. Patients with low levels of carnitine are more likely to suffer severe anemia that requires treatment with erythropoietin and more likely to have epoetin-resistant anemia, so supplementation with L-carnitine may be effective for some patients.

20. D: During hemodialysis, if a patient complains of chest pain, begins coughing, and shows evidence of cyanosis of the distal extremities and lips, the nurse should suspect that the patient has an air embolism. In the supine recumbent position, the air often enters the heart (as opposed to the brain if the patient is sitting upright), generating foam in the right ventricle and into the lungs. If air returns from the lungs to the left atrium and ventricle, it can enter the arterial system and cause severe cardiac and neurological impairment.

21. A: To prevent further complications, the nurse should immediately clamp the venous line and stop the blood pump to avoid the introduction of more air. Air emboli are usually venous although arterial emboli can occur. Hypovolemia and sitting upright during dialysis are risk factors because they reduce venous pressure. Air emboli may result from leaks in the circuit or air in dialysate solution. Air can also be introduced during insertion or removal of central venous catheters.

22. C: In response to these symptoms, the patient should be positioned in the Trendelenburg position on the left side or flat supine (depending on center protocol). Treatment is symptomatic and may include oxygen, intubation and ventilation, and cardiac catheterization or percutaneous needle insertion for aspiration of air from the atrium or ventricle. In some cases, treatment in a hyperbaric oxygen chamber may be utilized to prevent cerebral edema.

Section Description: Kim Case Questions

23. B: When evaluating a patient in preparation for creation of a fistula, the blood pressure difference between the arms should be less than 10 mm Hg. This is a normal finding. A difference of 10 to 20 mm Hg is a borderline finding, and a difference of more than 20 mm Hg is cause for concern. All upper extremity pulses should be assessed as well as pulse oximetry. The Allen Test should be carried out to assess circulation of the radial and ulnar arteries.

24. D: When conducting the Allen test to assess circulation of the radial and ulnar arteries, arterial insufficiency is indicated when the blanching persists for ≥5 seconds. For the test, the patient should extend the arm and hand, palm upward. The nurse compresses both the radial and ulnar arteries at the wrist while the patient pumps the hand repeatedly to help the hand to blanch. Once the hand is blanched, the ulnar artery is released and duration of blanching of the palm is noted. Then, all compression is released and the procedure is repeated for the radial artery.

25. B: For preoperative assessment of vessels, Doppler ultrasonography is often done under regional anesthesia of the arm because anesthesia causes the veins to dilate, making them easier to visualize and assess. Doppler ultrasonography is used to measure the inner diameters of the arteries and veins as well as the flow velocity. However, central veins cannot be adequately visualized with Doppler ultrasonography. The vein dilation and arterial dilation tests are done during Doppler ultrasonography as well as vein mapping.

26. B: Following a period of maturation, an AV fistula should have a diameter of at least 6 mm before it is used for hemodialysis. According to the "rule of 6s," the diameter should be at least 6 mm and the depth below the skin less than 6 mm. Additionally, a straight segment of at least 6 cm should be present and the AV fistula should accommodate a flow rate of at least 600 mL/min. This degree of maturation usually takes about 6 weeks but may extend up to 4 months in some patients.

27. C: When auscultating an AV fistula to listen for the bruit, if the nurse notes the bruit is very high pitched, this may indicate stenosis. The thrill should be low-pitched and constant. The other indications of stenosis include a pounding ("water-hammer") pulse, decreased thrill, intermittent bruit, edema of the access limb, increased venous pressure during treatment, recirculation, clotting of the extracorporeal system during treatment, excessive bleeding after removal of needles at completion of hemodialysis, "black blood syndrome," and decreased Kt/V and URR. Common sites for stenosis are inflow (juxta-anastomotic stenosis), outflow, and central vein.

28. D: When using the buttonhole technique for vascular access for hemodialysis, the needles are placed in the same sites in a fistula with one site for the arterial needle and one for the venous needle. KDOQI guidelines recommend teaching the patient to self-cannulate. The buttonhole technique cannot be utilized with a graft because the grafts lack muscle fibers to close the hole after the needle is removed. Using the same holes with a graft could result in a permanent opening and exsanguination.

29. A: When inserting a needle for hemodialysis, rotating the needle to any degree increases the risk of infiltration, and even one incidence of infiltration may damage an access. The nurse should be very gentle and proceed slowly when cannulating and should level the needle to the surface of the skin before advancing it. Using a wet needle reduces the risk of infection and makes observing for flashback easier. The needle should be gently flushed with NS after insertion to ensure it is placed properly.

30. A: If, following formation of an AV fistula, the nurse notes that the patient's nail beds and skin on the hand below the fistula are cyanotic during hemodialysis and the patient complains of pain in the hand, this is likely an indication of steal syndrome (AKA dialysis access-associated hand ischemia). The hand may feel noticeably cooler than the opposite hand. Steal syndrome may occur in up to 20% of accesses. Upper arm access increases risk of steal syndrome as does diabetes and peripheral arterial disease. Patients may complain of pain, paresthesia, and coldness of the hand during dialysis.

Description: Independent Questions, Group 1

31. D: The permeability of a dialyzer membrane to water is indicated by its ultrafiltration coefficient (K_{UF}). The ultrafiltration coefficient listed for a dialyzer indicates the amount of water that will pass through a membrane at a given pressure in a specified unit of time

(generally one hour). For example, if the K_{UF} is 10, then 10 mL of water will pass through the membrane for each mL of mercury (mm Hg) of transmembrane pressure. So if the transmembrane pressure were 100, then the patient would lose 1000 mL (10 X 100) of water each hour.

32. D: Dialyzers should be processed within 2 hours. If a dialyzer is to be reprocessed after more than 2 hours (such as in 3 hours), the dialyzer must be refrigerated because the cold helps to retard the growth of bacteria. The dialyzer must be refrigerated during any transportation to another facility for reprocessing. However, the dialyzer should not be frozen. The exact temperature is usually set by the manufacturer and/or the hemodialysis center.

33. A: Blood tubing for hemodialysis is generally color-coded to help decrease the chance of errors with arterial tubing color-coded red and venous tubing color-coded blue. Some types of equipment may require custom tubing sets for individual patients. Blood tubing includes patient connectors that connect the blood tubing segments to the patient's needles/catheter ports, dialyzer connectors that allow connection to the dialyzer, and drip chamber or bubble trap to check the arterial or venous pressure. The heparin and saline infusion lines are usually placed on the arterial tubing segment.

34. B: During hemodialysis, usually 100 to 250 mL of blood is outside of the patient's body at one time. However, if a separation of a bloodline occurs, much more blood may be lost in a small amount of time because the blood flow rate is usually set to pump between 300 and 500 mL per minute. This continuous flow, if undetected, could result in exsanguination. For this reason, it is imperative that the access site is open to view at all times and that the patient be carefully monitored during treatment.

35. D: When setting up a surveillance program for a hemodialysis center to monitor bloodstream infections (BSIs), once this event has been chosen for monitoring, the next step is to determine the time period for observation, such as a month, quarter, or year. If BSIs are rare, then a longer time period is indicated in order to ensure measurement validity. Then, surveillance criteria and data elements to be collected must be determined followed by outlining the method for data analysis and methods for data collection.

36. C: In order to increase absorption of iron for patients with chronic kidney disease on oral iron supplements, patients should be advised to take the supplement on an empty stomach because taking it with food may decrease absorption. Additionally, patients should avoid enteric-coated preparations and should not take the supplement with phosphate binders. Patients are usually prescribed 325 mg ferrous sulfate three times daily, as this is equivalent to 200 g of elemental iron daily.

37. D: According to the NHSN Dialysis Event Surveillance guide, the standardized infection ratio (SIR) is calculated based on the number of observed bloodstream infections (BSIs) divided by the number of predicted BSIs, based on national statistics and the number of patients. If the results show a SIR greater than 1.0, then the facility has a rate of BSIs higher than predicted. A score of 1.0 indicates the rate of infection is the same as predicted and an SIR of less than 1.0 indicates that the BSI rate is lower than that predicted.

38. D: Albumin is the molecule that has the highest molecular weight, calculated in daltons (Da): 66,000 Da. Dialyzer membranes screen for different molecular weights with the

molecular weight cutoff representing the molecule with the highest molecular weight able to pass through the membrane. Larger molecules have greater molecular weight. Creatinine has a molecular weight of 113 Da, urea has a molecular weight of 60 Da, and calcium has a molecular weight of 40 Da.

39. B: Backwashing to free residue from sediment filters in the water system should be done at least one time daily. Sediment filters strain residue, such as particles and solutes, from the feed water. The filters are layered with each layer screening out more and more particles, but the channels in the filter can plug if the sediment builds up, so the water flow through the unit is reversed to flush the sediment out of the filter. This process may be done automatically.

40. C: The usual dose of potassium in dialysate is 2.0 mM, although the dose may be increased to 3.0 mM if the patient experiences hypokalemia (<4.5). Patients on digitalis also require a higher dose of 3.0 mM. If this results in higher potassium levels between dialysis treatments, then patients may require routine administration of sodium polystyrene sulfonate resin (Kayexalate®). Utilizing potassium doses of 1.0 mM routinely to control hypokalemia is contraindicated because of increased risk of cardiac arrest.

41. A: If a physician has prescribed midodrine 10 mg for a patient to take 2 hours prior to hemodialysis, the most likely reason for this medication is to prevent intradialytic hypotension resulting from inadequate vasoconstriction. Contraindications to this drug include supine hypertension and active cardiac ischemia (although the drug may be administered with coronary artery disease without ischemia). However, if a cooler dialysate solution is being used to prevent intradialytic hypotension, adding midodrine does not provide increased benefit.

42. C: In order to reuse dialyzers, the dialysis center must follow standards developed by the Association for the Advancement of Medical Instrumentation (AAMI). CMS utilizes these standards as well under their conditions of coverage or ESRD facilities. Standards are set for both manual and automated reprocessing, but most reprocessing is done by companies that specialize in reprocessing because of the cost of equipment and the strict standards. All automated equipment must be approved by the FDA.

43. B: Prior to using a reprocessed dialyzer, a recirculating rinse with NS should be completed with recirculating flow rate through the blood compartment (BFR) of 200 mL/min and recirculating flow rate of 500 mL/min through the dialysate compartment (DFR). The rinse is carried out for a period of 15 to 30 minutes, being careful to avoid introduction of air into the arterial circuit, as air may interfere with the removal of germicide. Test strips are used to ensure all germicide is cleared from the dialyzer.

44. A: When influencing others to continuously improve practice, the nurse should recognize that the first step in the change process is to believe in the possibility of change. Without a positive frame of mind, the nurse is not likely to convince others that taking action will make a difference. Believing is following by making a decision to change and then taking action. Understanding the results of change is usually the last step in the process.

45. B: The best response to a new team member who is less productive than others on the interdisciplinary team and often finishes work late is to speak directly with the team member about the observations. There may be many reasons that a new team member is

less productive than others on the team, including insecurity, lack of knowledge, lack of experience, or poor time management. It often takes new team members time to achieve the same level of expertise as those with more experience on the team.

46. C: With the formula for urea kinetic modeling (UKM), the "K" in the Kt/V formula stands for urea clearance (mL/min) plus residual urinary output. UKM is one method of estimating the dose of dialysis delivered. The "t" refers to the duration of dialysis in minutes. The "V" refers to the volume of fluid in mL in the patient's body. This volume is not measured but is calculated by a computer program, and accurate volumes can be difficult to estimate.

47. A: During peritoneal dialysis, the concentration gradient of a substance, such as urea, decreases. That is, more urea diffuses into the instilled dialysate when the concentration is low than when the concentration increases. In order to compensate for this change in concentration gradient, more frequent exchanges can be done (such as is common with APD) or dwell volume may be increased, although this typically cannot exceed 2.5 to 3 L.

48. A: When considering interdisciplinary communication, the nurse's reporting on a patient's condition in a team meeting is an example of collegial communication (AKA inter-collegial communication). The three basic types of communication are social (chatting about vacation), therapeutic (answering a patient's questions and providing one-on-one instruction), and collegial (communicating with colleagues). Collegial communication may be in spoken form (such as reporting on a patient's condition) or written form (such as writing a summary of the patient's condition or problems).

49. A: The purpose of the peritoneal equilibration test is to determine the amount of glucose absorbed from dialysate and the amount of urea and creatinine filtered into the dialysate in a 4-hour dwell. This is one method of assessing the effectiveness of peritoneal dialysis. This test also helps to identify those with high rate of transport because these patients may rapidly absorb glucose and may need to have shorter dwell times. If the amount of urea and creatinine filtered is inadequate, the patient may need a longer dwell time or more exchanges.

50. A: Glucose in dialysate must be heat sterilized at low pH in order to decrease generation of glucose degradation products (GDPs), which can irritate the peritoneal membrane. For single-compartment dialysate bags, the dialysate is heated at 5.5 pH because a lower pH solution would be too painful for instillation. However, in a double-compartment bag, the glucose-containing dialysate is heat sterilized at about 3.2 pH, while the other compartment is heat-sterilized at an alkaline pH. Then, the two compartments are mixed before instillation.

51. D: The primary purpose of using an amino-based dialysate solution for PD is for nutritional supplementation as it promotes uptake of amino acids in skeletal muscles. However, the amino-based solution can only be used one time daily in order to prevent acidosis and increased serum urea levels. The solution is usually absorbed within 4 to 6 hours and is most effective if administered after meals to aid in protein synthesis. Amino-acid solution is osmotically comparable to 1.36% glucose.

Section Description: Walker Case Questions

52. C: If a hemodialysis patient's itching persists and the patient's Kt/V is 1.1, the dialysis adjustment should be to increase the Kt/V to greater than 1.2. The usual target is 1.4 to ensure that the patient's level doesn't fall below 1.2. Improving the quality of dialysis may, in some patients, relieve itching to some degree, although the evidence is not clear. Elevated calcium, phosphorus, and parathyroid hormone levels may also cause itching in some patients.

53. B: If adjusting a patient's Kt/V and changing dialyzers do not relieve itching, the intervention most indicated should be moisturizers and oil bath as dry skin is generally the most common cause of itching. High levels of phosphorus, especially, may cause itching. If emollients do not control itching, then antihistamines, such as Benadryl, or other treatments, such as ultraviolet lights or gabapentin, may be considered. Naltrexone or tacrolimus ointment may relieve severe and persistent itching.

Section Description: Chang Case Questions

54. C: For a patient with chronic kidney disease, education about the different options for renal replacement therapy should generally begin when the patient's GFR is equal to or less than 30 mL/min/1.73 m². Patients are often very stressed when dealing with the reality of dialysis, so they may be more receptive to education and better able to make a considered choice before their need for dialysis is imminent. Discussion should include different types of access (catheters, grafts, fistula) as well as different types of dialysis (CAPD, APD, home dialysis, nocturnal dialysis, in-center dialysis).

55. D: When teaching a patient about hemodialysis, the best way to determine that the teaching plan is geared to the patient's educational ability is to ask the patient directly about his or her educational background and preferred style of learning. While, for example, a person with an advanced degree may be able to understand more complex explanations than a high school dropout, this is not true for all people. When people are under stress, this can interfere with their ability to learn and to remember.

56. A: A disadvantage of hemodialysis compared to peritoneal dialysis is poor control of blood pressure, with the patient especially at risk for hypotension. Other disadvantages to hemodialysis include the need for heparin, which may increase the risk of bleeding, the need for vascular access, and the necessity of following a relatively strict diet. Peritoneal dialysis, on the other hand, increases the risk of obesity, peritonitis, hernia, malnutrition, hypertriglyceridemia, and back pain.

57. A: There are few contraindications to hemodialysis because it is used in life-threatening circumstances. However, hemodialysis is contraindicated if the patient exhibits hemodynamic instability, inability to coagulate blood, or if there is a lack of access to systemic circulation. Metabolic acidosis, changes in mentation, and hyperkalemia are all indications for hemodialysis. Other indications include fluid overload, elevated BUN (>90 mg/dL), elevated serum creatinine (≥9 mg/dL), drug toxicity, and signs of uremia. Hemodialysis is also indicated if there are contraindications to other forms of dialysis.

58. D: When teaching a patient about hemodialysis, the patient should understand that the primary advantage of short daily hemodialysis (at least 5 to 6 times weekly) is reduced left

ventricular hypertrophy, a common complication associated with chronic kidney disease and hemodialysis. Patients also experience improved physical functioning. These advantages hold true even if the total hours are similar to those of patients receiving hemodialysis in a center 3 times weekly for 4 hours. Short daily hemodialysis is usually done in-home rather than in a hemodialysis center.

59. C: Approximately 36 to 48 hours of peritoneal dialysis are equivalent to 6 to 8 hours of hemodialysis. Patients typically have 4 or 5 exchanges every 24 hours (often 3 to 4 during daytime hours and a longer one at night) with dwell times in the daytime typically averaging about 4 to 6 hours. Hemodialysis, on the other hand, is more commonly done for 3 to 4 hours 3 times weekly. Thus, hemodialysis is less time-consuming and requires less effort on the part of the patient, but the patient also may be more restricted in travel and less independent.

60. B: A history of diverticulitis is a contraindication to CAPD because the increased intra-abdominal pressure may result in rupture of the diverticulum. Other contraindications (not all absolute) include abdominal adhesions from previous surgeries, immunosuppressive drugs, colostomy, ileostomy, nephrostomy, or ileal conduit, and severe arthritis in the hands or impaired mobility of the hands. Inability to carry out the treatment independently is usually considered a contraindication. Patients who are legally blind or who have partial vision loss may be able to manage CAPD.

61. B: Patients with kidney disease considering the herpes zoster (shingles) vaccination should be advised to take 1 dose if age 60 or older in order to decrease the risk of developing shingles and decrease the severity of shingles should they occur. However, post-transplant patients or any other patient receiving immunotherapy should not receive the immunization because the herpes zoster vaccine is a live virus vaccine, and those with depressed immune systems may develop the disease if they take the immunization.

Section Description: Pham Case Questions

62. A: The patient is presenting with typical signs and symptoms of autosomal dominant polycystic kidney disease—enlarged kidneys, gross hematuria, and flank (or abdominal) pain. Diagnosis is per ultrasound, and criteria varies according to age, reflecting the fact that the number of cysts tends to increase over time:
- < 30: Two or more total cysts.
- 30 to 59: Two or more cysts in each kidney.
- ≥60: Four or more cysts in each kidney.

63. D: If a patient with autosomal dominant polycystic kidney disease has enlarged kidneys because of multiple cysts, the patient is most at risk for additional cysts in the liver. Hepatic cysts occur in up to one-half of patients with ADPKD. Cysts may also occur in the pancreas and spleen, but they are less common. The cysts are distinct from the relatively harmless cysts that develop in the kidneys associated with older age.

64. A: The gross hematuria associated with autosomal dominant polycystic kidney disease most often results from rupture of a cyst into the renal pelvis, especially as the cysts enlarge. However, in some cases, the hematuria may result from development of renal lithiasis or urinary tract infection. Bleeding usually recedes within a week of bedrest and adequate hydration. Persistent bleeding should arouse suspicion of renal cell carcinoma.

65. C: The type of kidney stone that is most likely to occur in a patient with autosomal dominant kidney disease is calcium oxalate. These kidney stones occur in about 1 in 5 patients. Hydration of 2 to 3 L of fluid daily is encouraged to help prevent formation. Foods high in oxalate should be limited, including chocolate, soy products, nuts, nut butters, blackberries, blueberries, raspberries, figs, kiwis, concord grapes, beans, beets, greens (collard, beet, kale, spinach, Swiss chard), squash, peppers, olives, and okra.

66. D: If a patient with autosomal dominant polycystic kidney disease and enlarged cystic kidneys develops sudden onset of excruciating pain in the lower back, right flank, and right abdomen, the most likely cause is bleeding in a cyst, causing it to rapidly expand in size. As cysts expand in size, the traumatized vessels stimulate angiogenesis, which in turn increases the risk of bleeding. If the bleeding is confined, the patient may not have hematuria. If the cyst ruptures, the patient may experience retroperitoneal bleeding and severe pain and/or hematuria.

Section Description: Jackson Case Questions

67. B: Anti-glomerular membrane glomerulonephritis (Goodpasture syndrome), an autoimmune disorder that destroys collagen in glomeruli and alveoli, is typically characterized by kidney failure and pulmonary hemorrhage, although about 33% of patients may not exhibit pulmonary injury. Goodpasture syndrome is more common in males than females and is most common in males in their teens or 20s. Kidney failure may occur very rapidly. The disorder is often preceded by a viral infection or exposure to toxins, such as hydrocarbon solvents.

68. A: The primary treatments for anti-glomerular membrane glomerulonephritis (Goodpasture syndrome) include plasmapheresis to remove the circulating antibodies and corticosteroids (or sometimes other drugs) to serve as immunosuppressive agents. Plasmapheresis is usually done daily for up to 14 days. Antihypertensives, such as ACE inhibitors and ARBs are usually provided to control hypertension in order to protect the kidneys. Patients who require dialysis often have poor prognosis.

Section Description: Independent Questions, Group 2

69. A: According to KDOQI guidelines, when administering hemodialysis to a patient, a facemask should be worn for all access connections. If patients are doing their own cannulations, they should be advised to also don facemasks. Strict aseptic technique and proper hand hygiene with soap and water and/or alcohol-based hand rub are also critical elements in preventing infections. Patients should be advised to monitor staff members for compliance and to insist staff wear masks and use appropriate techniques.

70. B: If two patients in the hemodialysis center are afebrile with no complaints at the onset of hemodialysis but begin to have chills and spike a fever with 45 to 60 minutes, the most likely cause is pyrogenic reaction. Pyrogenic reactions result from pyrogens such as bacterial toxins, and commonly affect more than one patient at the same time. If pyrogenic reaction is suspected, then the dialysis should be stopped. Whether or not the patient's blood is returned depends on center policy.

71. C: When inserting needles into a graft, the needle tips should be at least 2.0 inches apart. Needles should be inserted at least 0.5 inch away from previous needle sites and at least 1.5 inches away from the anastomosis or any sign of stenosis. The arterial needle is placed toward the arterial anastomosis and the venous needle toward the venous anastomosis (keeping a minimum of 1.5 inches away from the anastomosis). When inserting a needle, the nurse should always consider first where the needle tip will rest.

72. B: If a patient on hemodialysis exhibits a change in personality and increasingly aggressive and threatening behavior, the best response it to refer the patient for a psychiatric evaluation. About 1 in 10 patients hospitalized for end-stage kidney disease also have a psychiatric disorder, and these conditions may be precipitated or exacerbated by the stress of dealing with a chronic illness, functional and dietary restrictions, and sexual dysfunction. Patients who are on medications for psychiatric disorders may need to have medication protocols modified.

73. B: An 18-year-old patient is legally an adult and, therefore, may choose to discontinue treatment, and there is little recourse if the patient is of sound mind. Because the patient has agreed to stay on medications, the best response is to provide education and support, showing respect for the patient while acknowledging concern. The patient should be thoroughly apprised of signs of uremia, as the patient may change his mind when his condition deteriorates.

74. A: Peritoneal dialysate is rendered hyperosmolar with the addition of glucose. Dialysate usually contains sodium, chloride, and lactate or bicarbonate. Although alternate osmotic agents, such as icodextrin and amino acid solutions are available, glucose remains the most widely used, although it may result in patients absorbing 200 to 300 g of glucose daily. This may further result in hyperglycemia and weight gain because of the additional calories, as well as increase risks of hyperlipidemia and cardiovascular disease.

75. C: If a peritoneal dialysis patient with suspected hydrothorax is to have a radionuclide scanning with technetium, the patient should be advised to remain ambulatory after instillation and between scans so that intra-abdominal pressure is increased and the tracer enters the pleural cavity. A scan is usually taken immediately on instillation and then at 10-minute intervals (0, 10, 20, 30) for 4 scans. In some cases, another scan may be completed in 2 to 3 hours.

76. C: When a catheter is inserted for peritoneal dialysis, the length of the subcutaneous tunnel is usually 5 to 10 cm. The tunnel extends from the peritoneal cavity through muscle and subcutaneous tissue to the skin. The catheters usually contain a set of cuffs, with one cuff distal to the peritoneum and the other subcutaneously at least 2 cm from the exit. The cuffs hold the catheter in place, prevent leaks, and provide barriers that reduce the risk of infection.

77. B: Rigid non-cuffed catheters should be used for peritoneal dialysis for a maximum of 3 days, usually only for acute care. These catheters pose an increased risk of infection and should be avoided if possible, but one may be inserted before a chronic cuffed catheter to allow immediate dialysis. Rigid non-cuffed catheters are typically made of a semi-rigid plastic material and may be curved or straight. They are inserted with the use of an internal stylet that facilitates percutaneous insertion.

78. C: During the initial preoperative assessment with stencil-based mapping as part of planning for insertion of a peritoneal catheter, the surgeon applies the stencil to various places on the chest and abdomen to determine the optimal placement of the catheter. At this session, the surgeon usually only marks the exit site, but immediately before surgery, the surgeon may make more extensive markings, including at the incision area, the exit site, and the tunnel track to ensure proper placement.

79. D: The most common cause of impaired outflow with peritoneal dialysis is constipation. If the colon is full of feces, this may result in mechanical pressure that displaces the tip of the catheter or it may block the side holes, interfering with drainage. Bowel function should be monitored carefully and treated with an emollient (70% sorbitol solution, one ounce every 2 hours) until the constipation resolves. Urinary retention and distended bladder are less common causes of impaired outflow.

80. D: If a peritoneal catheter is placed but not used immediately, it should be irrigated within 72 hours to ensure patency. The irrigation is done with 1 L of normal saline or dialysate solution. The irrigation helps to remove blood or fibrinous material that may have collected in the peritoneum. The irrigation may be repeated if the effluent is very sanguinous. Following initial irrigations, the catheter should be irrigated weekly until in routine use for dialysis.

81. B: If a patient receiving peritoneal dialysis complains of discomfort at the exit site and the nurse notes that the subcutaneous cuff has extruded, the initial intervention is probably to shave the cuff using a scalpel. The extruded cuff can provide a reservoir for bacteria, which can then ascend the tube, so removing the cuff is essential to reduce the risk of infection. Catheter splicing, which is more difficult, may also be done in some cases.

82. C: According to KDOQI guidelines, Kt/V urea should be measured in patients after initiating peritoneal dialysis after one month of treatment and then every 4 months. Additionally, if there are any changes of note in the patient's condition or changes in the dialysis prescription (such as volume, duration, changes in dialysate, or additives to dialysate), the Kt/V urea should be measured. If patients consistently meet their target goals, some patients may have routine measures extended to 6 months.

83. B: According to NKF-DOQI clinical practice guidelines, peritoneal dialysis should be initiated when the Kt/V urea falls below 2.0 because of increased risk of malnutrition and uremia with lower values. This is especially important if the patient is exhibiting signs of malnutrition, such as decreased serum albumin or unintentional loss of weight. However, even with a Kt/V urea below 2, some conditions may be considered in delaying initiation, including stable weight, lack of edema, lack of clinical indications of uremia, and nPNA ≥0.8g/kg per day.

84. C: A symptom that is most specific for depression in a patient with uremia is repeatedly thinking about dying. While all of the other symptoms (changing patterns of sleep with insomnia, feeling tired and lethargic, and exhibiting psychomotor agitation) are also commonly found with depression, they are also common to uremia and can be mistaken for depression, which does frequently occur with uremia. Repeatedly thinking about dying or imagining committing suicide are always cause for concern.

85. B: The best time to discuss advance directives with a patient who is diagnosed with kidney failure is early after diagnosis when the patient is most likely to be able to think clearly and make a considered decision. Advance directives allow the patient to indicate preferences for end-of-life care if the patient is no longer able to do so. In some states, the advance directive may contain a durable power of attorney. However, in some states, the durable power of attorney is a separate legal document that indicates who can make healthcare decisions for the patient if the patient cannot.

86. D: The presence of organic material, such as blood or semen in the urine may give a false positive for a urine albumin dipstick. Other causes of false positives may include alkaline urine, radiocontrast agents, contamination with detergents or disinfectants, and urine specific gravity of greater than 1.030. False negatives are associated with specific gravity of less than 1.010, acidic urine, increased urine sodium, and presence of nonalbumin proteinuria.

87. D: The most common reason for resistance to therapy with an erythropoiesis-stimulating agent (ESA) is iron deficiency, which occurs in up to 40% of patients with chronic kidney disease and interferes with the action of the ESA. Resistance is defined as no increase in hemoglobin level one month after treatment with ESA. Because of the problem of resistance, iron levels should be assessed before beginning ESA treatment. ESA therapy is indicated when hemoglobin levels fall below 10 g/dL.

88. C: In order to slow the progression of chronic kidney disease in patients with chronic metabolic acidosis (usually associated with GFR of less than 25 ml/min/1.73^2), sodium bicarbonate should be administered to maintain the serum bicarbonate level at 22 mmol/L. It is important to control metabolic acidosis because it also results in increased reabsorption of bone, increasing the risk of fractures. The dose of sodium bicarbonate that is usually administered is 0.5 to 1.0 mmol/kg/day.

89. D: The primary difference between glomerular filtrate, the product of glomerular filtration, and plasma is that glomerular filtrate does not contain proteins. Filtrate contains water, amino acids, uric acid, electrolytes, glucose, urea, and creatinine. Plasma proteins are not filtered out of the blood because they are too large to pass through the glomerulus. Glomerular filtration is carried out through the process of ultrafiltration and requires adequate blood pressure as well as blood volume.

Section Description: Schwartz Case Questions

90. D: If a patient on peritoneal dialysis believes that increasing overall dwell time compensates for skipping peritoneal dialysis two days per week, then the patient does not understand some of the basic principles behind dialysis and needs re-education to ensure that he has a good understanding of the risks involved in skipping treatments. A fully informed patient is better able to make decisions. If the patient still wants to persist in having treatment-free days, then the patient may need to consider switching to hemodialysis.

91. A: While longer dwell times do often result in increased clearance of toxins, with excessive dwell times, a point of equilibrium is reached at which fluid and toxins no longer move and some effluent may be reabsorbed back into the body as the osmotic gradient is lost. Patients should be advised to discuss any change in schedule of dwells with their

nephrologists to ensure that the peritoneal dialysis is meeting the patients' needs and to prevent complications.

92. C: If a patient on CAPD initially had approximately 400 mL of residual urine daily but the volume has been decreasing, the patient will most likely need longer dwell times or larger volumes of dialysate. Residual kidney function is considered when prescribing peritoneal dialysate, but with a decreased urinary output, the patient's ultrafiltration rate to remove water must increase to compensate. The patient may also add additional exchanges or use dialysate with a higher concentration of glucose.

93. D: If a patient on CAPD complains frequently about quality of life issues (a common concern with patients on dialysis), the assessment tool that may be most appropriate is SF-36 (short-form health survey), which specifically assesses these issues. The method provides assessment in 8 areas: physical functioning, pain, role limitations associated with physical or emotional health, emotional status, social functioning, energy level, and general perceptions of personal health. This is a self-assessment tool that the patient can usually complete in less than 15 minutes.

Section Description: Locke Case Questions

94. D: If a 23-year-old female has recently started peritoneal dialysis and calls to report that she has noted a small amount of blood in the effluent, the first question to ask the patient is "Are you menstruating?" While blood in the effluent is not generally a normal finding, it may occur for the first few initial treatments until the tissue is well healed. Blood may also be evident during menstruation as the hypertonic fluid in dialysate can pull menstrual blood through the fallopian tubes and into the peritoneum.

95. A: Many patients are concerned about appearance when undergoing peritoneal dialysis and are worried about the kinds of clothing that they can wear. While there is some variation from one individual to another, the average waist size increases during treatment by only 1 to 2 inches. However, the catheter and any apparatus (tubing, bags) also take up space, so loose-fitting clothing is generally most appropriate. Some patients, especially those who are younger, may benefit from assistance of a fashion consultant.

96. D: If a patient who has started on peritoneal dialysis complains of a constant sweet taste in the mouth, the reason for this is probably absorption of glucose from dialysate. Some patients also develop a sweet aftertaste in their mouths after ingesting artificial sweeteners, such as aspartame. Patients may also complain of a metallic taste in their mouths, and this is often associated with the buildup of toxins in the blood between treatments.

97. D: If a patient on CAPD has been losing weight and becoming malnourished because her appetite is very poor and she feels full and slightly nauseated when she tries to eat a large meal, the initial best solution is probably to eat small, frequent meals. Patients often feel full because of increased intra-abdominal pressure created with dwell and may feel nauseated if they try to force themselves to eat more. Simply adding vitamin supplements is not adequate, as patients need calories as well.

98. A: If a patient's effluent shows many fibrin strands and clots that are interfering with outflow, the recommended treatment is the addition of heparin to the dialysate. Treatment with heparin should be initiated when the fibrin strands are first observed because if

obstruction occurs, irrigating with different solutions or with heparin is of little value. If the heparin is unsuccessful in improving outflow, then tPA instilled after NS irrigation is sometimes used to try to dissolve fibrin clots.

Section Description: Independent Questions, Group 3

99. B: If a patient is undergoing hemodialysis and the nurse notes that a bloodline has separated and blood has pooled beneath the access site, the first intervention should be to stop the blood pump and then to clamp both sides of the separated line to prevent further loss of blood. Both sides of the separated line are considered contaminated, so the line should not be reconnected, and the blood remaining in the line must be discarded.

100. B: If a pseudoaneurysm occurs in a fistula, the most likely cause is improper rotation of needle sites. A pseudoaneurysm occurs when the graft widens because of weakness of the wall. This may result from a defect related to too numerous punctures of the same site. Signs include swelling at the site, shiny and stretched skin, discoloration of the skin, and pain. Because the pseudoaneurysm poses a risk of rupture and exsanguination, the nurse should never insert a needle into a pseudoaneurysm.

101. D: If a patient who has had severe recurrent episodes of gout has recently started on hemodialysis, the patient should expect that the episodes of gout would decrease. Uric acid is a small molecule so it is filtered from the blood during hemodialysis. However, if overproduction of uric acid continues, the patient may still experience some symptoms of gout because the production may still exceed the removal. Patients may need to continue with a low purine diet.

102. C: If a diabetic patient with chronic kidney disease is rapidly deteriorating and is starting hemodialysis and the patient has taken high doses of insulin for many years, the insulin dosage will likely need to be decreased. Insulin is dependent on the kidneys for excretion, so with kidney failure, the insulin remains active in the body for longer periods. Additionally, some patients who had been insulin dependent are able to stop taking insulin with dialysis. Glucose levels should be carefully monitored and insulin dosage individualized.

103. B: Because the patient's hemoglobin (6.2) and hematocrit (19.1) are dangerously low, the nurse should initially hold the dialysis treatment until the physician responds. Continuing with the dialysis when the patient's blood counts are so low puts the patient at risk of cardiac arrest. The patient may require transfusions in order to increase the blood counts and may need more aggressive management of anemia with EPO and iron. The patient should be assessed for signs of bleeding.

104. C: Because pericardial effusions may suddenly enlarge and result in cardiac tamponade, surgical drainage is usually considered when the effusion volume exceeds 250 mL. The most common procedure is a subxiphoid pericardiostomy done under local anesthesia. If the effusion is less than 250 mL, increasing the frequency of dialysis to 5 to 7 times per week may resolve about half of the pericardial infusions. Medications such as NSAIDS and steroids have not proven to be helpful.

105. A: If a hemodialysis patient is experiencing severe anxiety, an appropriate medication is lorazepam, which is a short-acting benzodiazepine metabolized by the liver, although the

medication should be given for a limited period of time. Diazepam is contraindicated for those on hemodialysis. Barbiturates, such as phenobarbitol, are removed through dialysis and should not be used for anxiety. In some cases, such as when the patient becomes extremely agitated, haloperidol may be prescribed.

106. B: For a patient who has been treated for bacterial peritonitis with IP antibiotics, loss of protein may result in malnutrition as well as poor healing. The patient's diet may need to be adjusted to ensure adequate protein intake, and the patient should be monitored closely. Prompt diagnosis and treatment of peritonitis are essential in preventing malnutrition. Patients may present with malnutrition on diagnosis of peritonitis, and the condition is likely to worsen during the course of treatment, increasing the risk of mortality.

107. B: If a patient on CAPD plans to take a trip out of state and stay for a week in a hotel, the best advice to help the patient for the trip is to arrange to have supplies sent to the destination 2 to 4 weeks before arrival, contacting the hotel first to make sure they have storage space and to understand that a number of large boxes may arrive. The patient should also call a few days prior to arrival to make sure all of the supplies have arrived.

108. B: If a patient is switching from CAPD with a nighttime dwell to APD with daytime dwell, the adjustment in the procedure that is likely to result from receiving dialysis during sleep is an increased volume of dialysate for the nighttime dwells. In the supine position, there is less intra-abdominal pressure, so the abdomen can tolerate a larger volume of fluid. Typical dwells during the night are with 2 to 3L of dialysate while the daytime dwells are usually 1.5 to 2L. The number of exchanges may vary with CAPD and APD, although the nighttime dwells with APD are often of shorter duration.

109. A: If a patient on peritoneal dialysis has erythema about the exit site and purulent discharge although the dialysate solutions return clear, then the patient most likely has an exit site and possibly a tunnel infection. Because *Staphylococcus aureus* is a common bacteria found on the skin and is one of the most common causes of exit-site infection, empiric therapy that is started before the return of culture results should cover this organism. If the patient has previous history of *P. aeruginosa* infection, then the antibiotic should cover this organism as well.

110. C: With the post-dilution mode of hemodiafiltration, the blood goes through the hemodialyzer and then the fluid is added as it leaves the dialyzer, so the blood in the dialyzer is not diluted. This means that low-to-high molecular weight solutes are well cleared through convection. All or part of the fluid infusion can be done upstream of the filter if desired to bring about hemodilution, but this decreases the clearance of solutes.

111. A: If a diabetic patient receiving acute hemodialysis is hyperglycemic with glucose level of 270 mg/dL, the electrolyte imbalance of primary concern is hyponatremia because sodium levels decrease as glucose levels increase because of a shift of water from the intracellular compartment to the extracellular. Excess plasma is retained rather than excreted when the usual osmotic diuresis triggered by hyperglycemia does not occur, preventing correction of the hyponatremia. Administration of insulin to lower the glucose level causes the retained fluid to shift back to the intracellular component, correcting the hyponatremia.

112. B: If a patient scheduled for acute hemodialysis has a serum sodium level of 132 mmol/L, the initial goal should be to maintain the serum sodium level at ≥140 mmol/L. The dialysate solution should be less than 10 mM higher than the patient's serum sodium level, especially if the patient is at risk for hypotension or cerebral edema. If the patient's serum sodium level is less than 130 mmol/L, then the sodium level should be corrected slowly (6 to 8 mmol/L in 24 hours) in order to prevent severe neurological impairment.

113. D: If a patient is severely hyperkalemic with abnormalities noted on the ECG, including depressed P waves, peaked T waves, and widening of the QRS complex, the treatment that is most appropriate while the patient is waiting to begin acute hemodialysis is infusion of calcium chloride or calcium gluconate to bind to the potassium. Alternate treatments include administration of IV glucose and insulin or administration of inhaled or intravenous albuterol.

114. B: If a patient is involved in a sudden deceleration automobile accident and experienced a severe blunt injury to the abdomen and complains of severe abdominal pain and has hematuria, the preferred method of evaluating for renal trauma is with a CT scan because it can aid in accurately staging the degree of injury and can help identify any other abdominal injuries that may be present. With severe injury to the kidney, damage to other organs is a common finding.

115. D: In order to be a candidate for renal transplant, the patient's GFR usually must be equal to or less than 20 mL/min/1.73 m^2. Patients who want a preemptive transplant may want to be placed on the waiting list early, but time on the list is credited from the time the GFR falls to 20 mL/min/1.73 m^2. This GFR is categorized as stage 4 chronic kidney disease. Stage 5, kidney failure, occurs when the GFR falls to less than 15, the point at which the patient will require transplantation or dialysis.

116. A: While criteria may vary slightly from one transplant center to another, lack of financial resources or insurance to cover the costs of the transplant is usually considered an absolute contraindication because of the high costs associated with the procedure and immunosuppressive therapy that follows surgery. However, patients may be eligible for medical assistance through Medicaid, and Medicare covers transplantation. Additionally, the American Kidney Fund through the Health Insurance Premium Program may provide some financial support so that patients can pay for their insurance.

117. C: Patients should have a realistic understanding of the lifespan of a transplanted kidney. The average lifespan is 10 to 15 years; however, in actuality the expected lifespan for an individual kidney varies according to the age and condition of the recipient. Kidneys implanted into younger patients may last longer than 15 years, while a kidney in an older adult may only last 4 to 5 years. Many patients will require more than one transplanted kidney over their lifetime, especially if they received the first transplant as a child or younger adult.

Section Description: Rivera Case Questions

118. D: If a 68-year-old patient with diabetes, type 2, peripheral neuropathy, hypertension, and proteinuria has a serum creatinine of 1.7, then the patient should not be taking metformin because it may result in lactic acidosis when the serum creatinine reaches this level. Metformin is contraindicated for males with serum creatinine equal to or greater than

1.5 mg/dL or for females with serum creatinine equal to or greater than 1.4 mg/dL. Patients with kidney disease and taking metformin must be closely monitored.

119. A: If the patient's LDL level is 142, the goal of statin therapy and diet should be to decrease the patient's LDL to at least less than 100 mg/dL, although in some cases the goal may be set even lower, such as to below 70 mg/dL. The patient's LDL level is now categorized as borderline high (130 to 159 mg/dL). Because LDL is the primary cause of atherosclerotic plaques and arterial obstruction, it's important to lower the LDL level and increase the level of HDL, which functions to remove cholesterol and should be greater than 60 mg/dL.

120. A: Patients should be counseled to avoid strenuous exercise and red meat for 8 hours prior to a serum creatinine test, as these may interfere with the results. Serum creatinine indicates the kidneys' abilities to excrete waste. Normal values vary from one laboratory to another but are usually less than 1.2 mg/dL. Elevation of the serum creatinine is an indication of renal disease. Urine creatinine should always be considerably higher than serum creatinine.

121. C: When instructing a patient about preparation for an intravenous pyelogram (IVP), the patient should be advised to expect to have a bowel prep the day before the test as well be NPO for 8 hours prior to the procedure. The IVP is a fluoroscopic procedure that requires injection of a radiopaque dye and a series of radiographs. Following the IVP, the patient should be encouraged to drink fluids to help flush the dye and should be monitored for signs of allergic response.

122. A: Diabetic nephropathy results from damage to the glomeruli, which are part of the functioning unit of the kidney, the nephron. The nephrons comprise the renal corpuscle and the renal tubule. The filtering unit in the renal corpuscle is the glomerulus (a cluster of blood capillaries), and a sac-like structure that surrounds it, Bowman's capsule. With diabetic nephropathy, the glomeruli become scarred and are no longer able to adequately filter the blood of solutes. The first indication is often the finding of microalbuminuria.

123. D: When a patient is severely dehydrated and hypotensive, the hypertonic plasma that results stimulates the posterior pituitary to release ADH. ADH increases reabsorption at the renal tubules, decreasing urinary output in an effort to increase blood volume and to increase blood pressure. In response to hypotension, the kidneys release renin, which converts angiotensinogen (produced by the liver) to angiotensin I, which is in turn converted into angiotensin II by a lung enzyme. Angiotensin II is a vasoconstrictor that helps increase blood pressure.

Section Description: Williamson Case Questions

124. C: If a patient presents with sudden onset of hematuria, nausea, anorexia, severe left costovertebral angle pain, and tenderness in the left flank on palpation, the most likely diagnosis is acute pyelonephritis. Pyelonephritis, an inflammation of the renal pelvis, may affect one or both kidneys and is often the result of an ascending infection, such as cystitis. Chronic pyelonephritis may develop if the patient has longstanding or recurrent urinary tract infections, and this can lead to scarring of the kidneys.

125. B: The purpose of a nitrite production test is to evaluate for the presence of bacteria in the urine, specifically bacteria that produce nitrites, including *Escherichia coli, Klebsiella, Proteus, Pseudomonas, Salmonella, Citrobacter,* and some species of *Staphylococcus.* A negative finding, however, is not conclusive because negative results may occur when the patient has elevated specific gravity or is taking ascorbic acid. The nitrite production test will not detect the presence of pathogens that are non-nitrite-producing.

126. A: If a patient is treated for acute pyelonephritis in the ED with a dose of parenteral ceftriaxone and sent home with a prescription of ciprofloxacin 500 mg twice daily, the antibiotics are usually taken for 7 days. The duration varies according to the medication prescribed, but first-line antibiotics are usually given for shorter durations (5 to 7 days) than second-line therapies, such as TMP-SMZ, which is administered for 14 days. The choice of antibiotic should be influenced by resistance patterns in the local area.

Section Description: Bukowski Case Questions

127. D: While acute interstitial nephritis may occur as the result of infection or autoimmune disorders, such as Sjögren syndrome or systemic lupus erythematosus as well as electrolyte imbalances, such as hypokalemia or hypercalcemia, the most common cause is a reaction to drugs (7 out of 10 cases). The drugs that most often are associated with acute interstitial nephritis are cephalosporins, penicillins, sulfonamide-containing diuretics, rifampin, NSAIDs, phenytoin, and proton pump inhibitors. Infections associated with acute interstitial nephritis include CMV, histoplasmosis, streptococcal infections, leptospirosis, and Rocky Mountain spotted fever.

128. B: The blood abnormality that is a common finding with acute interstitial nephritis is increased eosinophils. This occurs in about 8 out of 10 patients. While prognosis is usually good, recovery may be a slow process lasting months, and about a third of patients will require temporary acute hemodialysis, although most will not progress to end-stage kidney disease. Identifying and removing the causative agent for drug-induced disease is critical to recovery. In some cases, patients may be treated with corticosteroids if they don't respond to supportive care.

Section Description: Robinson Case Questions

129. A: If a patient understands the necessary dietary restrictions, further consultation with a renal dietitian may not be of use. The most useful response is probably to refer the patient to a Meals on Wheels program. Most of these programs provide limited special diets, such as low sodium and/or low carbohydrate, and the choices are likely more nutritious than fast food. Costs are generally low, and many programs deliver a main meal in the middle of the day and include cereal for breakfast the next day and a snack for dinner.

130. D: The Confusion Assessment Method is a tool designed to determine if a patient is experiencing delirium. The 9 factors covered by the tool include the onset, attention level, thinking ability, level of consciousness, orientation, memory, perceptual disturbances, psychomotor abnormalities, and sleep-wake cycle. The tool is intended to be used by those without psychiatric training. Delirium is characterized by fluctuating symptoms. Various factors can trigger delirium, such as electrolyte imbalances and dehydration, putting patients with chronic kidney disease at risk. Delirium may be precipitated by uremic encephalopathy and dialysis dysequilibrium.

131. D: The task that is appropriate to assess a patient's ability to concentrate is to ask the patient to repeat the days of the week backward, to count backward from 100 by 7s, and to spell the word *world* backward. Patients may also be asked to carry out a simple three-part task (giving the directions one step at a time in case memory is impaired). When assessing intellectual ability and sensorium, the nurse should evaluate orientation, memory, and ability to think abstractly.

132. B: If an elderly patient with multiple co-morbidities has almost reached stage 5 chronic kidney disease, but the patient is not a candidate for transplantation and the patient's prognosis, even with dialysis, is very poor, the best solution is to discuss the prognosis and options with the patient so the patient can decide if he wants a trial of hemodialysis or prefers to opt for palliative care only. While family members may be included in the discussion, unless the patient is not of sound mind, the decision rests with the patient.

133. A: For a patient with non-dialytic chronic kidney disease and elevated PTH, the KDIGO guidelines recommend treatment with vitamin D. Hyperparathyroidism, a common finding with kidney disease, acts as a uremic toxin and may result in bone disease. The target PTH level varies with the type of assay used and will increase over time because of resistance to PTH that develops in the bones. After patients are started on dialysis, the target PTH range is usually 2 to 9 times the normal range.

Section Description: Independent Questions, Group 4

134. B: The most important consideration for patients in their approaches to health beliefs and health practices is usually cultural background. Non-Western cultures may view illness as caused by an unnatural force, such as a deity or spirit, or as caused by a natural force, such as heat or cold. Patients who consider the source of illness outside of themselves may not be receptive to changing personal behavior in order to treat or prevent illness.

135. C: If, prior to beginning treatment for diabetes, the patient's Hgb A1C was greater than 10%, a realistic target goal Hgb A1C for this patient is less than 7%. The patient will need to not only take medications but also modify his diet in order to achieve this response. Studies have shown that lowering the Hgb A1C in adults with chronic kidney disease to less than 6% increases the risk of mortality. If the patient's pre-diabetic baseline Hgb A1C is available, then the patient's target goal may be individualized to within 10% of normal.

136. B: For a patient at stage 4 kidney disease considering options, the patient should understand that the best survival rate is associated with pre-emptive transplantation. Pre-emptive transplantation is an especially good option if the patient is receiving a donated kidney from a family member or friend because the surgery can be planned for and scheduled in advance without concern that a kidney may not be available. Another advantage is that long-term costs are decreased; however, the patient must take long-term immunosuppressive drugs.

137. B: The three processes involved in production of urine are:
- Glomerular filtration: Ultrafiltration process that produces glomerular filtrate.
- Tubular reabsorption: Much of the filtrate is reabsorbed through diffusion back into the blood, including water, electrolytes, and other solutes. This process demonstrates the ability of the kidneys to concentrate urine.
- Tubular secretion: Potassium and hydrogen ions are secreted back into the urine from the blood to regulate potassium levels and the acid-base balance.

138. D: The normal ratio of BUN to creatinine is 2:1. Urea is the end product of protein metabolism, and the blood urea nitrogen (BUN) test determines the ability of the kidneys to excrete urea. BUN may elevate because of various factors, including high protein diet, dehydration, hemorrhage, and medications. Creatinine is produced as a waste product when muscle breaks down. Levels in the blood should be low and they should be elevated in the urine. If the blood level increases, then this indicates that the kidneys cannot adequately excrete waste products.

139. C: If a patient with a Foley catheter requires a 24-hour urine collection for the creatinine clearance test, the proper procedure to collect the specimen is to place the catheter bag in a container of ice so that the urine remains chilled and then to collect the urine every hour, placing the collected sample in a refrigerated container until the entire 24-hour collection is completed. The creatinine clearance test usually requires collection for 12 to 24 hours.

140. A: If a hospitalized patient who is incontinent of urine has undergone a renal scan, the nurse should wear gloves while handling the patient's urine and changing soiled linen. If the patient is not incontinent and is able to use the toilet, then no special precautions are needed. However, healthcare personnel and others who are pregnant should avoid the patient for 24 hours after the procedure to avoid exposing the fetus to radiation. The radiation dose is relatively small and is excreted rapidly.

141. C: If a patient with kidney failure is to be assessed for possible vesicoureteral reflux, the test most indicated to confirm VUR is the voiding cystourethrogram. This procedure requires insertion of a catheter into the bladder and instillation of contrast dye. The dye outlines the bladder contour and shows reflux. The patient is asked to urinate while radiographs are taken as this provides extra information about the patency of the urethra and the bladder tone, as impairment may result in reflux.

142. B: If, after kidney transplantation, a patient requires medications not covered by his insurance drug plan and the patient is concerned that he may have to sell his home to pay for the drugs, the best response is to refer the patient to a social worker. Dealing with the financial problems of a patient requires expertise in knowing what resources are available, including programs for which the patient may meet the requirements, such as Medicaid or Medicare disability.

143. D: If a 38-year-old patient will soon require dialysis but lives 2 hours from a dialysis center and wants to carry out home dialysis so she can continue working and avoid disrupting her daily activities but lives alone and has no one to assist her, the best option for the patient is probably APD. The patient is not a candidate for home hemodialysis because she would need someone to assist her. Because of the distance to the hemodialysis center,

peritoneal dialysis is likely a better choice, and APD would allow the patient to have minimal disruptions during the day.

144. B: African American males who are HIV-infected have the most risk of developing HIV-associated nephropathy (HIVAN) although it can occur in all groups, especially in individuals with CD4+ counts of less than 200 cells/mm^3 and a high viral load. Diabetes, hypertension, older age, and co-infection with hepatitis B or hepatitis C are also risk factors. Patients with HIV should have routine kidney function tests, as almost a third of patients will eventually develop some degree of abnormal kidney function.

145. B: Hepatitis B-related glomerulonephritis is commonly associated with membranous nephropathy. With membranous nephropathy, the small vessels and basement membrane of the glomeruli become inflamed and thickened, interfering with the ability of the glomeruli to adequately filter the blood and to reabsorb protein, so that large amounts of protein are excreted in the urine. The goal of treatment is to prevent the progression of kidney damage, but about 1 in 5 patients will progress to end-stage kidney disease over time.

146. A: With chronic kidney failure, vascular calcification results from hyperphosphatemia, which in turn results in hypocalcemia because as phosphate levels increase in the serum, calcium levels fall. The decrease in serum calcium stimulates the parathyroid glands to secrete increased PTH. With kidney disease, the body does not respond normally to PTH, so calcium leaves the bones, resulting in osteomalacia, and builds up in the vessels, causing calcification. Additionally, vitamin D, which is needed for the body to properly utilize calcium, is not metabolized normally.

147. C: Urine osmolality indicates the amount of solutes in the urine. If the kidneys are unable to adequately filter the blood and remove waste products, the urine osmolality decreases. While urine osmolality may vary from 250 Osm/kg to 900 Osm/kg, the average adult with normal intake and kidney function has a urine osmolality of 500 Osm/kg to 800 Osm/kg of water. Therefore, an osmolality of 300 Osm/kg indicates early kidney disease. As urine osmolality decreases, serum osmolality should increase.

148. B: The number of grams of urea that is produced and excreted in 24 hours is 20 to 30. Urea is formed in the liver from ammonia and is an end product of protein metabolism. If the urine urea value decreases, this means that the kidneys are not adequately filtering out urea, so this can indicate renal disease. Because urea is synthesized in the liver, a decrease can also indicate liver disease. Urea may also be reduced if a patient is on a strict, low protein diet.

149. D: A positive Chvostek sign is associated with hypocalcemia. If the patient's facial nerve is tapped at the masseter muscle of the jaw (1 cm inferior to the zygomatic process/2 cm anterior to the ear), this induces a spasm (tetany) of the facial muscles on the same side because of hyperexcitability of the nerve. Chvostek's sign may also be positive with hypomagnesemia and in those with respiratory alkalosis.

150. A: Antidiuretic hormone (ADH) (AKA vasopressin) is secreted in response to an increase in blood osmolality. ADH is secreted by the posterior pituitary gland. Blood osmolality tends to increase and fluid intake decreases, and this stimulates the release of ADH, which in turn stimulates the kidney to increase reabsorption of water in order to

stabilize the blood osmolality. If however, the patient has excess fluid intake, ADH is suppressed and more water is excreted by the kidneys, resulting in diuresis.

151. A: The kidneys regulate the acid-base balance by (1) reabsorbing bicarbonate and (2) excreting acid. Serum pH must be maintained between the narrow range of 7.35 to 7.45, and the kidneys have a critical role. Bicarbonate is reabsorbed primarily in the renal tubules. Acid is produced as the result of protein breakdown, and the accumulation of these acids in the blood lower the pH, increasing the blood's acidity. Normal kidneys excrete approximately 70 mEq of acid daily.

152. C: The most common cause of secondary glomerular disease is diabetic nephropathy. Both primary and secondary glomerular disease are leading causes of chronic kidney disease, but diabetic nephropathy and hypertension are responsible for approximately 70% of end-stage kidney disease cases with most diabetic patients also exhibiting hypertension. Other causes of secondary glomerular disease include amyloidosis, HIV-associated nephropathy, sickle-cell nephropathy, and collagen-vascular disease. Acute glomerulonephritis may also result in chronic kidney disease, but it is not common unless extensive damage to glomeruli occurs.

153. D: The three most common cardiovascular complications associated with chronic kidney disease are (1) hypertension, (2) congestive heart failure, and (3) pericarditis. Hypertension is the most common complication and occurs in almost all patients because of sodium and water retention. About 75% of patients beginning dialysis have already developed left ventricular hypertrophy. Pericarditis may develop as the result of retaining metabolic toxins. A pericardial friction rub and/or jugular venous distention may be evident along with decreased cardiac output.

154. C: If a patient who had been ambulatory has begun to use a wheelchair because of increasing weakness and lack of stamina, the best response is to refer the patient to a physical therapist for evaluation and rehabilitation. Patients often become increasingly sedentary, and this results in loss of muscle mass and weakness. The physical therapist may be able to assist the patient with strengthening exercises and with a regimen of exercises that may increase strength or prevent further deterioration.

155. D: If a patient with chronic kidney disease has started to make threats against a member of his family and states that he wants the person dead and plans to use a gun to kill the person, the responsibility is to warn the person to whom the threats are directed. This is one circumstance under which confidentiality can be breached. The patient should also be referred to a psychiatrist for evaluation and should be evaluated for uremic encephalopathy, which can result in bizarre behavior.

156. C: Infection with *Clostridium difficile* may lead to kidney failure primarily because of dehydration that can occur very rapidly because of diffuse diarrhea and loss of fluids. Because of repeated contact with healthcare facilities and personnel, patients with chronic kidney disease are at increased risk of developing infection with *C. difficile,* and this increases risk of further morbidity and mortality. Spores of *C. difficile* are highly infectious, so the infection can spread readily from one patient to another. Risk increases for those receiving antibiotic therapy.

157. A: If a patient with chronic kidney disease has developed increasing urinary incontinence and his caregiver requests insertion of a Foley catheter to make care easier, the primary reason to avoid a Foley catheter is because a catheter increases the risk of infection. Catheters pose a daily risk of infection of up to 7%. Foley catheter use should be limited to less than a week if at all possible and should not be used solely for incontinence unless the urine has caused severe skin breakdown.

158. D: The primary coagulopathy associated with chronic kidney disease is platelet dysfunction. Mild thrombocytopenia may be present, but of greater concern is an abnormal ability of the platelets to adhere and aggregate. Patients may exhibit purpura and petechiae and may have prolonged bleeding times, increasing the risk of bleeding with surgical procedures. If the patient's hemoglobin is less than 10 g/dL, increasing the hematocrit to at least 30% may decrease the risk of bleeding.

159. C: If normal intake of potassium is about 100 mEq (3900 mg) per day, the usual limit for potassium if a patient's GFR has fallen to 15 mL/min/1.73 m^2 (<10 to 20 mL/min) is less than 50 to 60 mEq (1950 to 2340 mg) per day. Patients should be provided comprehensive lists that provide potassium content in various types of foods and given instructions in calculating the correct intake and planning meals. Because hyperkalemia is a common problem with kidney failure, patients must understand the importance of potassium restriction.

Section Description: Brown Case Questions

160. D: If a uremic patient presents in the ED with anorexia, nausea, fatigue, altered mental status, and signs of pericarditis, including pericardial friction rub, immediate acute hemodialysis is needed to prevent cardiac tamponade. Pericarditis may occur in up to 10% of patients with uremia. Pericarditis often leads to pericardial effusion as vessels break, leading to cardiac tamponade and, in some cases, cardiac arrest, so rapid intervention to reduce the inflammation associated with uremia is critical.

161. B: If a patient requires acute dialysis and has a serum urea level of 130 mg/dL, the initial target urea reduction should be <40%. In order to achieve this level, the blood flow rate should be set low to 150 to 200 mL/min, depending on the size of the individual. The initial hemodialysis session should be limited to 2 hours. These restrictions are important to prevent the development of disequilibrium syndrome, which can occur if blood solutes are removed too quickly.

162. A: When a venous catheter is inserted into the femoral vein for acute hemodialysis, the tip of the catheter should extend to the inferior vena cava as this location improves flow and prevents recirculation. The length required is about 20 cm. While use of the femoral vein is usually discouraged, it does have the advantage of being easy to access without risk of pneumothorax or hemothorax. Although the risk of infection is about the same as for other sites, risks include arterial puncture and retroperitoneal bleeding.

Section Description: Torres Case Questions

163. B: If a patient developed sepsis as the result of a urinary tract infection, causing acute kidney injury (AKI) and the need for CVVH, the maximal dose of dialysis is 25 mL/kg/hr, as higher rates have not been shown to reduce mortality rates or to improve the rate of

recovery. It is important to identify kidney injury as soon as possible and to institute early renal replacement therapy as any delay increases the risk of death. Use of citrate rather than unfractionated heparin results in better outcomes.

164. C: In order to avoid puncture of the carotid artery when a venous catheter for acute hemodialysis is placed in the right internal jugular vein of a patient with sepsis, the best preventive is use of ultrasound for guidance during the procedure. The veins of the neck may exhibit a range of variability, so use of anatomic landmarks may not be sufficient. In some cases, the carotid arteries may also be atypical, increasing the risk of carotid artery punctures and hematoma.

Section Description: Whitlow Case Questions

165. A: If a patient exhibits signs of renal artery stenosis (refractory hypertension, pulmonary edema, acute kidney injury, bruit over site of transplant), screening procedures may include ultrasound or MR angiography, but confirmation requires angiography. Renal artery stenosis is the one of the most common vascular complications of kidney transplant with symptoms usually occurring 3 to 24 months after transplantation. Complications of angiography are not common but can include bleeding at insertion site, perforation of the artery, thrombosis, and arterial dissection.

166. C: Risk factors for development of renal artery stenosis following kidney transplantation include cytomegalovirus infection, surgical trauma, fibromuscular dysplasia, and arterial disease with atherosclerosis a primary cause of renal artery stenosis. Other risk factors include the use of a pediatric donor kidney and delay in function of the donated kidney after surgery as well as lifestyle issues, such as inactivity, obesity, and smoking. One or both renal arteries may be affected. Renal artery stenosis is most common in males over 45 and in females over 55.

167. B: After confirmation of advanced renal artery stenosis, the treatment of choice is most often transluminal angioplasty with or without placement of stents. The stenosis may recur in about 1 out of 10 patients, and patients are at risk of acute rejection. If the stenosis is less than 50% and the patient is stable without significant deterioration of kidney function, the patient may be managed conservatively with medications. If angioplasty procedures are unsuccessful, then revascularization may be indicated.

Section Description: Abramov Case Questions

168. B: If a patient has received a deceased donor kidney, the information about the donor that can be shared with the recipient is the donor's age, gender, and race. The recipient cannot be told the donor's location, name, or address. If the recipient wants to contact the donor's family, the recipient can write an anonymous letter that will be forwarded to them. While some recipients have managed to track down a donor family, some donor families may not be receptive, and doing so is a violation of privacy.

169. D: Mycophenolate mofetil (MMF) is classified as an antiproliferative and is often used in maintenance therapy after kidney transplantation. Other antiproliferatives include azathioprine and sirolimus. MMF inhibits the activation of lymphocytes by preventing their proliferation. Patients must be carefully monitored for adverse effects, which can include infections and malignancies. Nausea and GI disturbances are common. Blood tests should be

monitored for leucopenia and thrombocytopenia, which can increase the risk of infection and bleeding. MMF is usually administered in oral form.

170. C: Core needle biopsies are usually done under ultrasound guidance, although the biopsies can also be done with CT, but CT-guided biopsy is more expensive and exposes the patient to radiation. Core needle biopsies are done with special 18-gauge core biopsy needles. The patient may receive conscious sedation as well as a local anesthetic while in the supine position. The core biopsy is usually obtained from the lower pole of the kidney.

171. A: If a patient is confirmed through renal biopsy as having acute rejection, the initial treatment is usually high doses of corticosteroids to depress the immune system. If the patient does not respond adequately to the steroids, then monoclonal antibodies, such as OKT3 or basiliximab are administered. In some cases, high doses of an antiproliferative agent, such as mycophenolate mofetil (MMF) may also be administered. Different centers use different protocols, but treatment may be individualized depending on patient response.

172. B: If a patient on immunosuppressive drugs following kidney transplant develops hand tremors, back and abdominal pain, somnolence, loss of memory, and dark urine as well as increased serum creatinine and BUN, the medication that is most likely responsible is cyclosporine. The increased blood pressure, hand tremors, somnolence, and loss of memory are especially indicative of cyclosporine. The cyclosporine level should be evaluated and will probably indicate toxicity. Cyclosporine levels are often taken daily until the optimal dose is established.

Section Description: El-Amin Case Questions

173. C: Early steroid withdrawal (after one week) following kidney transplantation is most associated with acute rejection, although steroid withdrawal is not associated with increased graft loss or death. Protocols differ from one center to another. KDIGO guidelines suggest one week of steroids and withdrawal or long-term steroids if initially given for longer than a week, but some centers give steroids for 2 weeks or even 3 months and then withdraw them. Early withdrawal of steroids decreases the risk of steroid-associated conditions, such as hyperlipidemia and diabetes.

174. A: With kidney transplantation, therapy with basiliximab is primarily used to prevent T-cell replication (which in turn prevents activation of B cells) and organ rejection. It is most often used as an induction therapy, given initially immediately prior to transplantation. Other induction therapies include thymoglobulin, OKT3, and daclizumab. While induction therapy targets T-cells, it also affects other cells and increases the risk of infection, so induction therapy is often given along with antimicrobials to reduce risk.

175. B: If following hospital discharge a week after a kidney transplant, the patient who had been doing well has sudden onset of fever of 38.8 °C, chills, tenderness about the incision, headache, and cloudy urine, the most likely cause is infection. The incision should be examined carefully for any drainage or signs of redness. Infections may be superficial or internal, so the patient should be advised to immediately report signs of infection to the physician because immunosuppression increases risk of severe infection.